Y0-AGT-485

Handbook of Common Poisonings in Children

Second Edition

Author: Committee on Accident and Poison Prevention
American Academy of Pediatrics

Regine Aronow, M.D., Editor

American Academy of Pediatrics
P.O. Box 1034
Evanston, Illinois 60204

COMMITTEE ON ACCIDENT AND POISON PREVENTION
1979-1983

H. James Holroyd, M.D., Chairman

Regine Aronow, M.D., Editor   H. Biemann Othersen, Jr., M.D.
Lorne K. Garrettson, M.D.   Barry H. Rumack, M.D.
Joseph Greensher, M.D.   J. Rafael Toledo, M.D.
Leonard S. Krassner, M.D.   Mark D. Widome, M.D.
Matilda S. McIntire, M.D.

Liaison

Andre l'Archeveque, M.D., Canadian Paediatric Society
Jerry Foster, M.D., American Academy of Pediatrics Section
on Emergency Medicine

Library of Congress Catalog No. 82-072740

ISBN No. 0-910761-03-5

Quantity prices on request. Address all inquiries to:
American Academy of Pediatrics
P.O. Box 1034, Evanston, Illinois 60204

©1983 by the American Academy of Pediatrics. All rights reserved.
Printed in the United States of America.

CONSULTANTS

The Committee wishes to express its appreciation to the following individuals for their valuable assistance and expert advice:

Walter R. Anyan, Jr., M.D., New Haven, Connecticut
J. Julian Chisolm, Jr., M.D., Baltimore, Maryland
Ralph E. Kauffman, M.D., Detroit, Michigan
Howard C. Mofenson, M.D., East Meadow, New York
Daniel C. Postellon, M.D., Detroit, Michigan

Contents

Tables

INTRODUCTION

The response to the *Handbook of Common Poisonings in Children* was so favorable that the Committee on Accident and Poison Prevention felt it worthwhile to update and revise it. Apparently, this book filled the gap between current handbooks on poisoning and texts on toxicology.

The items covered in the previous edition were taken from the National Clearinghouse for Poison Control Centers statistics of the 100 most common poisonings. Topics included in this edition are based on that list plus some serious poisons that require significant, therapeutic decisions. This edition deals primarily with topics by generic name. Two products are listed by trade name because they are widely used, and perhaps best known under the trade names.

The discussions are written to assist in the evaluation of the severity of the poisoning and to aid therapeutic decisions. Therefore, they are similar to therapeutic protocols developed by regional poison control centers.

Whenever possible, practitioners should check with regional poison control centers because therapeutic approaches to therapy tend to change. Some toxicants lack a medical consensus on the most appropriate treatment. Mixtures of poisons produce therapeutic quandaries, and the unique condition of the patient may contraindicate "standard" treatment. Few physicians have sufficient experience with the more severe or uncommon poisons to rely entirely on personal experience.

General Management of Acute Poisonings

The first and most important principle in dealing with a child who has been poisoned or is suspected of having been poisoned is to treat the patient not the poison. The physician or other medical personnel first encountering the child should organize a "team" effort. The most skilled team member should assess the patient's condition. Other team members should obtain a history, call the poison control center, and consult toxicologic resources. The person(s) directly in charge of the patient should attend to any need for an airway, respiratory assistance, circulatory support, or control of seizures.

If poison was spilled on the patient, promptly remove it or

dilute it with water, and remove contaminated clothing using gloves and other barriers as required to protect medical personnel. Contaminated clothing should be placed in an impervious bag and labeled. If poison is in the eyes, immediately irrigate them with isotonic saline, Dacriose solution, Ringer's lactate, or water; check for and remove contact lens, then, for 5 to 15 minutes, flush the eyes with the lids held open. Whenever a caustic has contaminated the eyes, irrigation should continue for at least 30 minutes, or until the patient is seen by an ophthalmologist. All strong alkali exposures require careful ophthalmologic examination. Absence of pain or complaint is an insufficient index of injury.

If the poison was inhaled, the patient should first be moved to uncontaminated air, and the rescuers should take precautions to avoid being overcome also. Adequate respirations and oxygenation should be maintained.

All substances that may be needed later for analysis, such as soaked clothing, vomitus, urine, and the noxious agent, should be saved in appropriate containers.

If the toxic substance is identified, specific directions for therapy should be provided by the "team member" who obtains the toxicologic information.

History

When taking the history about possible toxins, establish what each substance is used for, approximately how long ago it was obtained, and, if it is an uncommon substance, the name and address of the manufacturer. If a medication container does not list the name of the drug, record the prescription number and name and address of the store so the pharmacist can be asked specific details about medication, dose, and the amount prescribed.

Also, it is important to determine whether the patient has chronic health problems, which medications the patient may routinely be taking, and what medications were taken in the preceding 48 hours. Determine when and what food was eaten last.

The amount of substance ingested is established, when possible, by pill count or volume measurement and calculation from the amount present prior to the poisoning. When exact amounts of a substance are not known, the maximum possible dose should be used as a guide. Patients should be observed and/or treated as if the maximum dose was taken until the clinical course or laboratory measurements suggest a lower dose was involved. If two small children shared a toxin, proceed as if the smaller child has consumed the total missing amount. When liquids are consumed, it is useful to consider the "average size of a swallow:" 1½- to 3½-year-old child, 4.5 ml; adult female, 17 ml; adult male, 21 ml.[1]

Emesis

Emesis induced by Ipecac Syrup is the most efficient, rapid method to empty the stomach. Its active ingredients are cephaeline and emetine. They must be absorbed and carried to the medulla to be effective.

Ipecac Syrup should be given in the following doses: 1 to 10 years, ½ oz or 15 ml (1 tablespoon or 3 teaspoons); >10 years, 1 oz or 30 ml (2 tablespoons or 6 teaspoons). The dose has not been established for infants 1 month to 1 year old; 10 ml may be given, but it probably should be administered only in a medical facility under observation.

Follow Ipecac Syrup by one or two glasses of water. Some recommend 15 ml/kg of water, but care must be taken not to introduce a volume that may cause the pylorus to open. Milk is not recommended, except in special situations, because it delays the onset of vomiting following administration of Ipecac Syrup and makes it more difficult to identify the poison in the gastric content. The emesis should always be collected in a basin or pan so it can be inspected for the ingested material.

Emesis should not be attempted in patients who have lost their gag reflex, are convulsing, are in a coma or comatose condition, or have ingested a caustic (either acid or base). Some experts advise against emesis when the patient is having severe respiratory distress, when a substance such as camphor or strychnine may cause early convulsions, or when a substance such as liquid methadone may cause a quick onset of central nervous system depression. The ingestion of petroleum distillates is no longer considered a contraindication to emesis. Petroleum distillates appear to enter the lungs during deglutition. Unless an unduly large amount (greater than 1 ml/kg) has been ingested or a toxic agent is dissolved in the petroleum distillate, it is probably more judicious not to attempt emesis. If a toxic agent is dissolved in the petroleum distillate, emesis should proceed without delay,

---

1. Jones, D.V., and Work, C.E.: Volume of a swallow. Amer. J. Dis. Child., 102:427, 1961.

unless the patient is having severe respiratory distress or central nervous system depression.

If a pregnant woman ingests a dangerous substance, it may also be dangerous to the fetus. No recognized increment in toxicity to the fetus is added by the use of Ipecac Syrup to induce emesis.

Charcoal

Powdered, activated charcoal is an effective adsorbent of many toxins. Although it is more efficacious for some substances than others, activated charcoal may be used for all ingested materials except alcohols, lead, ferrous sulfate, boric acid, cynanide, DDT, N-methyl carbamate, malathion, mineral acids, and alkali caustics, or where it may interfer with specific, oral therapy of the poison—as in acetaminophen overdose. The usual dose of activated charcoal is approximately 8 to 10 times the ingested amount of poison, or between 10 and 30 gm. During the acute phase of some poisonings when gastric secretion of the agent (as with amphetamines) or excretion through the bile occurs (as with PCP, carbamazine, or tricyclic antidepressants), doses of activated charcoal every 4 to 6 hours are advisable.

Activated charcoal is administered as a slurry in water. (It should not be mixed with milk or ice cream because these decrease its efficacy.) The slurry should be kept stirred during drinking. It may be accepted more readily if it is iced and taken through a straw.

Activated charcoal should not be given concurrently with Ipecac Syrup because it will prevent the emetic from being absorbed, but activated charcoal does not bind saline laxatives (sodium or magnesium sulfate).

Only USP activated charcoal powder should be used. Tablets are not satisfactory as an adsorbent for poisons.

Gastric Lavage

Gastric lavage may be required to empty the stomach in patients who have lost the gag reflex, are having severe respiratory distress, have depressed sensoriums, or may convulse momentarily. Positioning the patient's head down, and preferably on the left side, helps prevent aspiration and allows for a greater return of gastric content. If endotracheal intubation is necessary in a small child before lavage, a snug-fitting tube, rather than a cuffed tube, should be placed by a person expert in this procedure.

The initial contents removed from the stomach should be saved separate from the rest of the gastric returns for possible analysis. The stomach should be washed with a tepid, half-strength isotonic saline solution until the return is clear, unless a specific lavage solution is indicated.

Note: If alkali caustics have been ingested, lavage should not be attempted. Cautious lavage within an hour of ingesting a strong acid may be indicated.

If the ingested material is in the form of tablets, capsules, or solids, the largest possible gastric tube should be used. In young children, this will be a 12- or 16-gauge tube. In older children or adults, a 32- or 36-gauge tube should be used. If many pills were ingested, a chemical bezoar may form. Radiopaque materials (such as chloral hydrate, heavy metals, iron, phenothiazines and enteric coatings) may be seen on an x-ray of the abdomen.

Dilution

After caustic ingestions, cautiously test swallowing competency with water. Dilution with a few swallows of water or milk may then be useful for caustic as well as irritant ingestions. Milk is not advised if endoscopy is anticipated.

Catharsis

Although decontamination of the lower gastrointestinal tract has only limited scientific proof of efficiency, it should be considered when solid materials are ingested, especially if enteric-coated tablets or delayed-release forms have been ingested. In the latter types of ingestions, saline cathartics are the agents of choice and cause catharsis osmotically. They may be given with or after activated charcoal.

Use sodium sulfate USP (Glauber salts), 250 mg/kg, or magnesium sulfate USP (Epsom salts), 250 mg/kg. For a toddler, the convenient approximate dose is: Glauber salts, ½ teaspoon (3 gm) in 1 oz of water, **or** Epsom salts, ½ teaspoon (3 gm) in 1 oz of water. Age 5 to 10 years, 2 teaspoons (10 gm) in 4 oz of water. Adults, at least 15 gm.

If no release of bowel content occurs in 4 to 5 hours, a rectal suppository may be used to start action.

Cleansing the Skin

If the poison is on the skin or clothing, the absorbed dose can be limited by prompt removal. Personnel handling the patient should wear gloves. Contaminated clothing should be removed and separately bagged.

The skin should be washed with soap and a copious amount of water. Tincture of Green Soap is preferable if it is available because some noxious substances dissolve better in alcohol. Give special attention to washing the umbilicus, hair, axilla, finger-nails, and genitals. Scrubbing is not necessary in the early phase of washing because it may remove the stratum corneum, which is the main barrier or rate-limiting step in absorption.

Poison in the Eye

Quick action is required when potentially toxic substances are in the eye. Washing out the toxin with tepid water must start immediately. After initial flushing with the eyelids held open, contact lens should be removed and the irrigation continued for at least 15 minutes. In the medical facility, isotonic solutions (saline, Ringer's lactate, Dacriose solution) should be used. Afterward, fluorescein may be used to evaluate the globe.

Any patient whose eyes were exposed to a caustic, or who has observed or suspected corneal damage, should have an appropriate referral for examination by an ophthalmologist.

Techniques of Monitoring

The monitoring of a patient for the development of symptoms or signs following an ingestion may be expedited by a flow sheet on which pertinent observations are recorded at predetermined intervals. Although different toxins require different sets of observations, appropriate observations should be established as soon as contact with the patient is made and the possible toxins identified. Flow sheets may be established by emergency medical personnel, nursing personnel, or medical staff.

Approximately one third of children will be drowsy after

administration of Ipecac Syrup, and it may be advisable to keep them from going to sleep until they are able to retain clear liquids.

Assessment of sedation is frequently difficult because a natural need for sleep occurs at nap time or night. Although it is rarely useful to keep a patient awake for a prolonged period of time, it may be necessary to awaken a patient at ½- or 1-hour intervals.

Pupillary size is best measured by a small hand ruler held in front of the eye. The amount of light must be the same at the time of each measurement.

Cardiac monitoring equipment should be used for patients involved in poisoning by any compound that may cause arrhythmia, hypoxia, hyper- or hypotension, and so forth. A common example is an overdose of a tricyclic antidepressant. With this type of poisoning, palpation and auscultation may be required every 5 minutes, or more frequently, and cardiac electronic monitoring is advisable.

Referral and Transfer

The decision to refer a patient depends on three factors: (1) the physician's knowledge of the toxin and/or his time constraints, (2) the required hospital facility for adequate care, and (3) the need for specialized laboratory support.

When decisions are required about antagonist use and the timing and size of repeat doses, a pediatrician more experienced in the care of poisoned patients or a medical toxicologist may need to be consulted. Telephone consultation frequently will be sufficient, and this should be freely sought through the regional poison control center.

Laboratory support usually can be obtained from regional laboratories, and the specimen rather than the patient can be transported. This is reasonable with specimens for diagnosis. However, if multiple specimens need to be drawn to monitor care (e.g., after methanol or ethylene glycol ingestion – when both toxin and therapeutic ethanol levels must be monitored), it may be best to transfer the patient.

Patients who require specialized monitoring may need to be transferred to appropriate centers. This is most apparent when continuous electrocardiogram, blood pressure, venous pressure, or central nervous system pressure monitoring is required. Appropriate respiratory support for the young child also may require transfer. Pediatricians in doubt about the need for specialized medical and/or nursing support should consult with a physician in the regional poison control center.

Telephone Contact

Most physicians or emergency personnel make their first contact with a poisoning episode through a telephone call. When taking a call, always initially obtain the telephone number and name of the caller so contact can be reestablished if the connection is interrupted. If the history is taken over the phone, the parent should be asked to read the label(s) on the substances. Establish what each substance is used for, approximately how long ago it was obtained, and, if it is an uncommon substance, record the name and address of the manufacturer. If a medication container does not list the name of the drug, record the prescription number and name and address of the store so the pharmacist can be asked for specific details on the medication, dose, and amount prescribed. Also, it is important to determine if the patient has chronic health problems, which medications the patient may routinely be taking, and what medications were taken in the preceeding 48 hours. Determine when and what food was eaten last.

With an estimate of dose, knowledge of the toxin ingested, and some information about the unique state of the patient, the physician must determine the appropriate therapy. Many first aid measures can be instituted at home if the ingested substance can be reliably identified. The child may require only observation at home, or decontamination, or single therapy; an office visit for medical evaluation, observation, or decontamination; an emergency room visit because of the potential for serious symptoms requiring medical evaluation, laboratory assessment, intensive therapy and/or admission.

If transport is required, give advice about the mode of transportation and exact details about where to take the patient (e.g., not just the emergency room, but the emergency room of Children's Hospital at street number and name).

Remind the caller that, if Ipecac Syrup is given prior to departure or if convulsions, coma, or airway obstruction might occur, an attending adult must accompany the driver and patient. Careful, safe driving to the medical facility should always be advised, and the caller should be reminded to bring the drug or toxin in its container and any vomitus, urine, or other identifying substance with them.

If the patient remains at home (which occurs in about 85% of inappropriate exposures), follow-up telephone contact may be advisable. Calls at 1, 4, and 24 hours after ingestion are appropriate in many instances. When poisoned patients are treated via phone, a sequential record of the event and the follow-up calls assure completeness (see sample form). Every toxic ingestion should be reported to the regional poison control center.

Poisoning Contact Form

Patient name: Date:

Phone number: Age:

Time initial call: Weight:

Suspected poison: Symptoms:

History of ingestion: Recent medication use—
                               general health:

Phone/office therapy:

Follow-up call time:

Referred to Hospital   Yes____No____Time_____

Referred to Poison Center Yes____No____Time_____

Referred to Toxicologist   Yes____No____Time_____

Copy of this form sent to poison control center:

Date_____

Prevention

The time of a poisoning incident, particularly when the incident is one of nontoxic ingestion or there are only mild or moderate symptoms, renders parents remarkably receptive to counseling in prevention. They have just learned "it can happen to me." Furthermore, large poison control centers now recognize that 85% of early childhood ingestions result in no significant illness. Thus, five of six incidents present a time when no therapeutic intervention is required, and consultation can be used to plan household accident prevention.

When a patient is cared for exclusively by telephone, the best time for prevention counseling comes on a call-back when observation has assured a favorable outcome, the parent is relieved and more relaxed, and the setting has changed from acute family perturbation that may have set up the psychologic environment and even precipitated the poison incident. During hospitalization, whether short term for observation or long term for therapy, the discussion of prevention is best near the time of discharge.

In all homes in which children less than 5 years old are cared for, a bottle of Ipecac Syrup should be kept handy for use **only** on medical advice from a physician or poison control center. If Ipecac Syrup is available for prompt administration (when it is not contraindicated), it may prevent an ingestion from becoming a poisoning. Ipecac Syrup in 1 oz bottles is readily available at pharmacies and some fast-food stores.

One inappropriate ingestion can occur in any family. Repeat episodes suggest a disorganized household; repeater children suggest a disruption in the mother-child relationship and deserve special counseling.

On occasion, the circumstances of a poisoning are suspect enough that a home visit by trained medical personnel is advised. Referrals should be made to public health nurses, social workers, police, fire departments, or other agencies for support when necessary.

Poison prevention counsel is an appropriate part of anticipatory guidance for all children. A good time to include it is at 9 months of age. At this time the parent is given or encouraged to purchase a bottle of Ipecac Syrup. Information to be shared with the spouse on poison proofing the home may also be given. The American Academy of Pediatrics includes poison prevention in TIPP (the injury prevention program). Suggested office tools for physicians are available from the American Academy of Pediatrics.

General References

The following reference list contains books likely to be useful for many different poisons. The reference materials needed will vary for each physician, depending on the type of practice, proximity to hospitals, and the availability of a regional poison control center and consultants in toxicology. For obvious reasons, the Committee recommends this *Handbook of Common Poisonings in Children.* The *Handbook of Poisons,* by Dreisbach, contains many useful tables and lists. Although some practitioners will wish to own the more comprehensive *Clinical Toxicology of Commercial Products,* many will prefer to rely on the services of the regional poison control center for more comprehensive reviews. With these comments, this list is offered.

Books

Arena, J.M.: Poisoning: Toxicology, Symptoms, Treatments, ed. 4. Springfield, Illinois: Charles C Thomas, 1979.

Dreisbach, R.H.: Handbook of Poisoning, ed. 10. Los Altos, California: Lange Medical Publishers, 1980.

Goodman, A.G., Gilman, L.S., and Gilman, A.: The Pharmacological Basis of Therapeutics, ed. 6. New York: Macmillan Publishing Company, Inc., 1980.

Gosselin, R.E., Hodge, H.C., Smith, R.P., and Gleason, M.N.: Clinical Toxicology of Commercial Products, ed. 4. Baltimore: Williams and Wilkins, 1976, reprinted 1977.

Haddad, L.M., and Winchester, J.F.: Clinical Management of Poisoning and Drug Overdose. Philadelphia: W.B. Saunders, 1983.

Hamilton, A., and Hardy, H.L.: Industrial Toxicology, ed. 4, revised by Finkel, A.J. Littleton, Massachusetts: John Wright/PSG, Inc., 1983.

Hardin, J.W., and Arena, J.M.: Human Poisoning from Native and Cultivated Plants, ed. 2. Durham, North Carolina: Duke University Press, 1974.

Hayes, W.J., Jr.: Pesticides Studied in Man. Baltimore: Williams and Wilkins, 1982.

Grant, W.: Toxicology of the Eye, ed. 2. Springfield, Illinois: Charles C Thomas, 1974.

Morgan, D.P.: Recognition and Management of Pesticide Poisonings. Washington, D.C.: U.S. Government Printing Office, 1982.

Physicians' Desk Reference for prescription and nonprescription drugs.

Microfilm System

Rumack, B.H., ed.: Poisindex, Englewood, Colorado, Micromedix Inc., 1982.

Laboratory Tests

Laboratory Tests for Office Use

Following are two tests that may be useful in the office by supporting historical and physical impressions, although they are not specific, are subject to false-negative results, and are not quantitative.

Lab Tests for Office or Clinic

Reagent	Preparation	Conduct of Test	Use
$FeCl_3$ 5%	5 gm of $FeCl_3 6H_2O$	Boil urine and cool. Add equal parts of reagent and urine. Dilute if too dark to assess color.	Salicylate gives purple color with gastric contents or urine. Some phenothiazines give red, orange, purple, or maroon color.

Once color develops, a few drops of strong acid into the solution will cause color due to salicylates to disappear. The color will remain if it was caused by phenothiazines (a phenostix will give a purple to brown color reaction with both phenothiazines and salicylates and cannot be used to differentiate between them).

| Deferoxamine | Add 4 ml distilled water to 1 ampule (500 mg/ampule) deferoxamine. | Place 2 ml gastric content in each of two plastic tubes. Add two drops of 30% H_2O_2. Add ½ ml deferoxamine to one tube. | Up to 3 hr after suspected iron ingestion, a light orange to dark red color confirms the presence of iron. |

Laboratory Tests in the Emergency Room

Laboratory tests help in three ways:

1. Assay of blood, gastric content, or urine may identify an unknown toxin or confirm that a toxin is involved in the illness.

2. Measurement of the concentration of toxin in the blood can, in some instances, indicate that the degree of illness observed is compatible with the level of toxin or that other toxins should be sought.

3. For a few toxins, serum levels will assist in predicting the future development of toxicity and the need for energetic, specific therapy before life-threatening symptoms develop.

When specimens are sent to laboratories for screening assays for unknown toxins, the toxicologist should be told what the physician suspects, what drugs were available, or what the clinical findings are, particularly when there are few leads to the toxic substance.

The laboratory values which are used to predict future toxicity may indicate the course of therapy. Serum or blood assays should be considered essential in most cases of poisoning with the following compounds: salicylates, acetaminophen, methanol, lead, mercury, arsenic, iron, ethylene glycol (rarely available), digitalis preparations, ethanol, barbiturates, phenytoin, theophylline, lithium.

Consult the local laboratory for specimen size, handling, and other assays which are available.

Urine screens are the most universally helpful. The physician should be aware of the actual substances included in the screen and the level of sensitivity of the tests. Some substances like LSD, lithium, and phencyclidine analogues will not be identified by these methods. Urine for heavy metal screens must be collected in specially prepared containers and specifically requested.

Drugs Used in Poisoned Patients

Formulary for the Office Management of Poisoned Patients

A small number of drugs may be useful in the treatment of mild poisoning or because time is short and treatment must begin before the patient is transported. Appropriately sized laryngoscopes, endotracheal tubes, gavage and lavage tubes, and equipment for ventilatory support is not listed but should be available (see p. 141).

Ipecac Syrup	Oxygen
Activated charcoal	Diazepam
Mg or $Na_2 SO_4$ (Epsom or	50% Glucose
Glaubers salts)	
Naloxone	Ethanol
Atropine	Epinephrine
Diphenhydramine	Amyl nitrate perles
Pyridoxine	BAL

Formulary for Emergency Room or Clinic Treatment of Poisoned Patients

A formulary of important drugs for the management of poisoning begins on p. 141.

Toxicity Calculations

Following are some calculations that may be of help in the management of poisoned patients.

The Anion Gap

Anion Gap is $Na - (Cl + HCO_3)$;
Normal range, 8 to 12 meq/l.

References:

Oh, M.S., and Carroll, H.J.: The anion gap. New Engl. J. Med., 279:814, 1977.
Emmett, M., and Narins, R.G.: Clinical use of the anion gap. Medicine, 56:38, 1977.
Done, A.K.: The toxic emergency. Emerg. Med., 12:145, October 15, 1980.

The Osmolar Gap

$$Osm \ (calc) = 1.86 \ Na + \frac{Glucose}{18} + \frac{BUN}{2.8}$$

Measured osmolality by freezing-point depression minus calculated osmolality = osmolar gap.

$$\Delta \, Osm = Osm \, (measured) - \frac{Osm \, (calc)}{0.93}$$

(Measures Osm expressed as mOsm/kg H_2O. Serum water approximately 93%.)

References:

Glasser, L., Sternglanz, P.D., Combie, J., and Robinson, A.: Serum osmolality and its applicability to drug overdose. Amer. J. Clin. Path., **60**:695, 1973.
Smithline, N., and Gardner, K.D., Jr.,: Gaps: Anionic and osmolal. J.A.M.A., **236**:1594, 1976.

Blood Ethanol Levels

The following formula can be used to predict the blood ethanol level after a single ingestion by a nonalcohol-dependent person:

$$c_p = \frac{dose}{V_D \times body \; weight}$$

c_p = plasma concentration in mg/l

dose = milligrams of ETOH

specific gravity of ETOH is 0.790 so 1 ml 100% ETOH = 790 mg

V_D = volume of distribution in liters per kilogram body weight

V_D ethyl alcohol:
   adult = 0.6 l/kg
   child = 0.7 l/kg

body weight = weight of patient in kilograms

Note: See Ethyl Alcohol (p. 68) for alcohol content of beverages. The same formula can suggest the dose of ethyl alcohol needed to achieve a given blood ethanol level, such as 100 to 150 mg/dl (mg%) in methyl alcohol or ethylene glycol ingestions.

Example: $1,000 \text{ mg/l} = \dfrac{\text{Dose (in mg)}}{V_D \text{ (in l/kg) x weight (kg)}}$

Blood ethanol level of 1,000 mg/l = 100 mg/dl (mg%) so dose (mg) = 0.6 (adult) x kilograms body weight x 1,000. Divide dose in milligrams by 790 to obtain milliliters of 100% ethanol required.

Ethanol is metabolized at the rate of approximately 125 mg/kg per hour in a nonalcohol-dependent person with normal liver function. To maintain a specific blood ethanol level after the loading dose, an infusion rate of approximately 125 mg/kg per hour is needed. **The first maintenance dose should be given concurrent with the loading dose.**

If dialysis is instituted, the clearance of ethanol requires an adjusted dose.

Another approach for calculating doses for ethanol therapy is:

Use 10% w/v ethanol in D_5W for intravenous administrations.

Loading dose: adult, 7.5 ml/kg; child, 8.75 ml/kg. Hourly dose: adult, 1.25 ml/kg per hour; child, 1.25 ml/kg per hour.

Infuse a sum of the first hourly dose and the loading dose over the first hour. Check blood alcohol level at 2 hours. The goal is to achieve a level of 100 to 150 mg/dl. Dialysis will increase the dose a variable amount, depending on the efficiency of the dialysis system. These doses are starting values. Great variation between patients requires individualization of the ethanol dose.

References:

McCoy, H.G., Cipolle, R.J., Ehlers, S.M., Sawchuk, R.J., and Zaske, D.E.: Severe methanol poisoning. Application of a pharmacokinetic model for ethanol therapy and hemodialysis. Amer. J. Med., **67**:804, 1979.

Peterson, C.D., Collins, A.J., Himes, J.M., Bullock, M.L., and Keane, W.F.: Ethylene glycol poisoning. Pharmacokinetics during therapy with ethanol and hemodialysis. New Engl. J. Med., **304**:21, 1981.

Harmon, W.E., and Sargent, J.A.: Ethanol during hemodialysis for ethylene glycol poisoning. New Engl. J. Med., **305**:522, 1981.

The Nontoxic Ingestion

Nontoxic ingestions are not true poisoning and can be adequately handled with simple reassurance by a poison information center or a knowledgeable physician. A nontoxic ingestion is the consumption of a nonedible product that usually does not produce symptoms. No product or drug is entirely safe; all can produce undesirable effects if ingested in sufficient concentrations or amounts.

The knowledge of the nontoxic ingestion serves to avoid overtreatment, placing the patient in jeopardy of a panicky automobile ride or the unnecessary use of emergency transport. It also serves as a warning of inadequate supervision or improper and unsafe environment and the potential of future, more serious ingestions. Knowledge of substances with a low toxicity potential allows us to recommend the least toxic effective product for use in the home.

The designation of "nontoxic" requires the following criteria:
1. absolute identification of the product,
2. absolute assurance that there was only one product ingested,
3. assurance that there is no signal word on the container,
4. reliable approximation of the amount ingested,
5. assurance that the patient is free of symptoms,

Table 1
Warning Labels

Following are the two systems of labeling for toxic substances in use in the United States today. These labeling systems are currently under review and may change.

Category	Label/Signal Word	LD_{50} Oral (mg/kg)	Household Measure
Household and Commercial Products			
1	No label	15 gm/kg	—
2	No label	5-15 gm/kg	ounce to pint
3	CAUTION	0.5-5 gm/kg	ounce to pint
4	WARNING	50-500 gm/kg	teaspoon to ounce
5	Danger: Poison	5 to 50 mg/kg	taste to teaspoon
6	Danger: Poison	<5 mg/kg	taste
Pesticides*			
1	Danger: Poison	<50 mg/kg	taste to teaspoon
2	WARNING	50-500 mg/kg	teaspoon to ounce
3	CAUTION	0.5-5 gm/kg	ounce to pint
4	No label	>5 gm/kg	pint or more

*Based on Insecticide, Fungicide, and Rodenticide Act of 1947.

Table 2
Frequently Ingested Products
That Are Usually Nontoxic

Abrasives
Adhesives
Antacids
Antibiotics
Baby product cosmetics
Ballpoint pen inks
Bathtub floating toys
Bath oil (castor oil and perfume)
Bleach (less than 6% sodium hypochlorite)
Body conditioners
Bubble bath soaps (detergents)
Calamine lotion
Candles (beeswax or paraffin)
Caps (toy pistols, potassium chlorate)
Chalk (calcium carbonate)
Clay (modeling)
Colognes
Contraceptives
Corticosteroids
Cosmetics
Crayons (marked A.P., C.P.)
Dehumidifying packets (silica or charcoal)
Detergents (phosphate only)
Deodorants
Deodorizers (spray and refrigerator)
Elmer's Glue
Etch-A-Sketch
Eye makeup
Fabric softeners
Fertilizers (if no insecticide or herbicides added)
Fish bowl additives
Glues and pastes
Golf ball (core may cause mechanical injury)
Grease
Hair products (dyes may be caustic; sprays, tonics)
Hand lotions and creams
Hydrogen peroxide (medicinal 3%)
Incense
Indelible markers
Ink (black, blue—non-permanent)

Idophil disinfectant
Laxatives
Lipstick
Lubricant
Lubricating oils (lipoid pneumonia)
Lysol brand disinfectant (not toilet bowl cleaner)
Magic markers
Makeup (eye, liquid facial)
Matches
Mineral oil (unless aspirated)
Newspaper (chronic may result in lead poisoning)
Paint, indoor, latex
Pencil (lead-graphite, coloring)
Perfumes
Petroleum jelly (Vaseline)
Phenolphthalein laxatives (Ex-Lax)
Play-Doh
Polaroid picture coating fluid
Porous-tip ink marking pens
Prussian blue (ferricyanide)
Putty (less than 2 oz)
Rouge
Rubber cement
Sachets (essential oils, powder, talc aspiration)
Shampoos (liquid)
Shaving creams and lotions
Soap and soap products
Spackles
Suntan preparation
Sweetening agents (saccharin, cyclamates)
Teething rings (water sterility)
Thermometers (mercury)
Thyroid tablet (dessicated)
Toilet water (alcohol)
Toothpaste (with and without fluoride)
Vaseline
Vitamins (with or without fluoride)
Warfarin (under 0.5%)
Water colors
Zinc oxide
Zirconium oxide

6. ability to maintain contact with the parent at intervals to determine that no symptoms have developed.

Table 3
Nontoxic House and Garden Plants

Plant identification is extremely difficult; but, if the caller can identify the plant and it is on this list, simple observation is advised. However, plants are foreign bodies and may be aspiration and digestive hazards.

African violet (Saintpaulia sonantha)
Aralia false (Dizygotheca elegantissima)
Begonia (botanical name)
Boston fern (Nephrolepis exata)
Christmas cactus (Zygocactus truncactus)
Coleus (botanical name)
Dandelion (Taraxacum sp)
Donkey Tail (Sedum organianum)
Dracaena (species)
Hawaiian Ti (Cordyline terminalis)
Hen and chicks (Escheveria or Sempervivum tectorus)
Honeysuckle (Lonicera sp)
Hoya (botanical name; wax plant)
Jade plant (Crassula argentea)
Lipstick plant (Aeschynanthus lobbianus)
Marigold (Tagetes sp and Calenduala officinalis)
Monkey plant (Ruella makoyana)
Mother-in-Law Tongue (Senservieria trifasciata)
Peperomia (botanical name)
Piggy-back plant (Tolmiea menziestii)
Pilea (botanical name)
Pink polka dot plant (Hypoestes sanguinolenta)
Plectranthus (botanical name)
Prayer plant (Maranta neuconeura kerchoveana)
Rose (Rosa sp)
Rubber plant (Ficus elastica; may cause dermatitis)
Schefflera (Brassaia actinophylla)
Sensitive plant (Mimosa pudica)
Snapdragon (Anterrhinum majus)
Spider plant (Anthericum or Chlorophytum cosmosum)
Swedish ivy (Plectranthus australis)
Violet (Viola sp)
Wandering jew (Zebrina bendula)
Weeping fig (Ficus benjamina; may cause dermatitis)

The designation of a nontoxic ingestion requires exact historical data and product identification. The information obtained should allow the questioner to feel confident that products other than the designated one have not been ingested, and to be reasonably certain about the amount ingested.

The average volume of a swallow of a 1½- to 3-year-old child is 4.5 ml, and of an adult it is 17 to 21 ml. This may allow an estimation of the amount ingested when the ingestion has been observed. It is difficult to define a large amount.

A "rule of thumb" for the toxicity of the average drug is that five times the therapeutic dose may be a toxic dose. A documented single tablet of most medications, even in an adult dose, will not produce significant toxicity if ingested by a child. Narcotics are an exception; an ingestion of narcotics requires medical examination and careful observation because the margin of safety is narrow, especially with Lomotil (diphenoxylate).

The emetic property of the ingested substance is important. Because rodents do not vomit, the rodent LD_{50} may be invalid to apply to humans when this defense mechanism in humans

Table 4
Nontoxic Berries

Common Name	Botanical Name	Color of Berry (season)
Pyracantha*	Pyracantha cocainea	Red (autumn and winter)
Dogwood, flowering	Cornus florida L.	Red (August and November)
Nandina	Nandina domestica	Red (summer and autumn)
Barberry	Berberis sp	Orange-red (autumn) Tan-spotted (winter)
Acouba	Acouba japonica	Red (autumn)
Mountain ash	Serbus auckpardia	Orange (later summer and autumn)
High cranberry	Viburnum opulus	Red (late summer and autumn)

*May have more poisonous varieties.

and other animals is overlooked. A systemic toxic dose of a detergent (anionic phosphate type) probably was not ingested if emesis has not been induced by the toxic agent.

The type of packaging may help determine whether a toxic amount could have been ingested; spray aerosol containers, pump containers, squeeze tubes, and so forth rarely produce a toxic ingestion.

The label and signal word is a clue to the toxicity of the product. If the label has "Danger, Poison," an antidote statement, or "Call Physician Immediately," the product may be toxic. Any label on the container stating "Danger, Poison," "Warning," or "Caution," automatically removes the product from the category of a nontoxic ingestion. The warning "Keep Out of Reach of Children" has no significance because many products with minimal toxicity carry this label. The current systems of warning labels are given in Table 1.

Any symptom, even if it appears unrelated to the ingestion, should exclude diagnosis of a nontoxic ingestion without a medical examination.

Exclude from consideration any nontoxic ingestions by children more than 5 years old. Ingestions by older children frequently indicate an intolerable home situation, and the child may require medical and psychiatric evaluation. These ingestions frequently are a "cry for help" and may represent a suicide attempt.

Examples of some nontoxic substances are given in Tables 2, 3, and 4.

Poisons

Acetaminophen

Type of Product: Analgesic, antipyretic.

Ingredients/Description: Acetaminophen is supplied in tablets of 80, 120, 325, 500, and 650 mg. It is also available in many cold and analgesic mixtures. Liquid acetaminophen preparations are also available in strengths ranging from 60 to 500 mg per 5 ml. The exact product name must be checked for acetaminophen concentration.

Toxicity: Acetaminophen is primarily hepatotoxic, and liver failure may result. An acute toxic dose of acetaminophen is considered to be 140 mg/kg. Unique patient factors, however, may influence this. There appears to be an undefined chronic toxic dose.

Symptoms and Findings: There are no unique signs or symptoms in the first 24 hours after an acetaminophen overdose to make the diagnosis definite. A patient who has ingested an overdose may exhibit generalized malaise, nausea, vomiting, and drowsiness. A latent period of 24 to 36 hours, which may progress up to 5 days, may occur between ingestion and onset of hepatic symptoms, with associated, elevated liver enzymes, elevated bilirubin, and disturbances in clotting mechanisms. Transient renal damage may occur after these changes.

Treatment: Induce emesis (Ipecac Syrup, p. 3) or perform a gastric lavage (p. 4). Activated charcoal should not be used because it interferes with the actions of the oral antidote, N-acetylcysteine (NAC). The need for definitive treatment should be based on an acetaminophen blood level taken within 24 hours of ingestion, optimally at 4 to 6 hours (see Nomogram defining possible hepatotoxicity). A 4-hour plasma level of 200 μg/ml is toxic, and the patient must be treated with NAC within 24 hours of ingestion. If the time of ingestion is unknown but estimated to be within 24 hours, two blood levels taken at least 2 hours apart may be used to calculate the half-life of the drug in the patient (see Table

SEMI-LOGARITHMIC PLOT OF
PLASMA ACETAMINOPHEN LEVELS VS. TIME

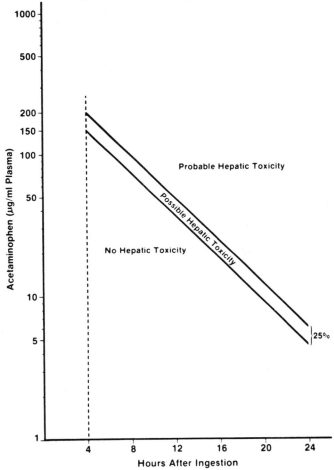

Rumack-Matthew Nomogram for acetaminophen poisoning. Cautions for use of this chart: (1) The time coordinates refer to time of ingestion. (2) Serum levels drawn before 4 hours may not represent peak levels. (3) The graph should be used only in relation to a single, acute ingestion. (4) The lower solid line 25% below the standard nomogram is included to allow for possible errors in acetaminophen plasma assays and estimated time from ingestion of an overdose. (Adapted from Pediatrics, 55:871, 1975, with permission from the authors and the publisher.)

Table 5
Acetaminophen Overdose*

To estimate half-life from serial blood levels†

% Decrease in Level Between Specimens	Multiply Time Interval by:
4	17
6	12
8	9
10	7
12	6
14	5
16	4
18	3.5
20	3
25	2.5
30	2
35	1.6
40	1.4
50	1
60	0.8
70	0.6
80	0.4
90	0.3

*If the actual time of ingestion is unknown but can roughly be estimated to be at least 4 hours earlier, two accurately timed blood levels can be used to calculate the half-life. It is a bad prognostic sign if the time of ingestion exceeds 4 hours. The hepatic injury appears to occur during the first pass of the drug through the liver. Adapted from Done, A. K.: Toxic emergency, Emerg. Med., 9:220, January, 1977.

†Example: If an initial level of 100 mg/dl drops to 80 mg/dl in 4 hours, half-life is about 3 x 4 = 12 hours.

5). If the half-life exceeds 4 hours, the risk of hepatotoxicity is probable, and definitive treatment is indicated.

Two agents have been successfully used for specific treatment of acetaminophen ingestion in this country. NAC (20% Mucomyst) has been used experimentally on a protocol from the Rocky Mountain Poison Center in the following dosage regimen: dilute a loading dose of 140 mg/kg 20% Mucomyst 4:1 with water, a cola drink, or fruit juice and immediately administer orally. This loading dose should be given as soon as possible after ingestion of the acetaminophen, but not later than 24 hours. The loading dose is followed by 17 additional oral doses of 70 mg/kg in the recommended dilution given at 4-hour intervals. Any dose of NAC vomited within 1 hour after administration should be repeated. If the episode involves a mixed overdose and activated charcoal has been given, lavage out the activated charcoal before giving NAC. If the results of blood levels absolutely are not available within 24 hours of the time of ingestion and the history indicates 140 mg/kg of acetaminophen has been taken, therapy should be instituted until laboratory results are available.

In the rare instances when the condition of the patient does not allow for oral administration of NAC, it may be diluted in D_5W and put through millipore filters for intravenous administration.

Methionine has been used in three different dosage schedules, but only if **within 12 hours of ingestion**: 100 mg/kg, intravenously, loading dose, then as a continuous intravenous drip every 8 hours for 3 days; oral dose — adults, 2.5 or 5 gm, orally, every 4 hours, repeated four times.

If more than 24 hours has passed since ingestion and a toxic dose was taken, monitor liver and renal function at least daily for 5 days and maintain the patient on a regime for impending liver failure.

References:

Peterson, R.G., and Rumack, B.H.: Pharmacokinetics of acetaminophen in children. Pediatrics, 62:877, 1978.

Peterson, R., and Rumack, B.H.: Toxicity of acetaminophen overdose. J. Amer. Coll. Emerg. Phys., 7:202, 1978.

Rumack, B.H., and Peterson, R.G.: Acetaminophen overdose: Incidence, diagnosis and management in 416 patients. Pediatrics, 62:898, 1978.

Committee on Drugs: Commentary on acetaminophen. Pediatrics, 61:108, 1978.

Prescott, L.F., Sutherland, G.R., Park, J., Smith, I.J., and Proudfoot, A.T.: Cysteamine, methionine, and penicillamine in the treatment of paracetamol poisoning. Lancet, 2:109, 1976.

Crome, P., et al.: Oral methionine in the treatment of severe paracetamol (acetaminophen) overdose. Lancet, 2:829, 1976.

Acetone

Type of Product: Solvent.

Ingredients/Description: Acetone is a colorless, volatile, and inflammable liquid. It has a characteristic aromatic odor and a pungent, sweetish taste. It is widely used in industry as a solvent for resins, plastics, cellulose acetate, lacquers, varnishes, rubber cement, glues, and nail polishes. A familiar use is as a nail polish remover.

Toxicity: Acetone has a relatively low toxicity. It is absorbed by ingestion, inhalation, and slowly through the skin. It is excreted mainly by the lungs (40 to 70% of an oral dose) and the kidneys (15 to 30%). Human adults given oral doses of 15 to 20 gm of acetone daily for several days showed no ill effects other than slight drowsiness.

Symptoms and Findings: The effects of acetone are similar to ethyl alcohol for equal blood levels, but the anesthetic potency is greater. Exposure to high vapor concentrations (e.g., 9,000 ppm) causes eye, nose, and throat irritation, restlessness, headache, vomiting, hematemesis, ketosis, fatigue, central nervous system depression, incoordination, stupor, and coma. Ingestion of large amounts produces the same symptoms. No serious systemic sequelae have been reported. Prolonged skin contact may produce dermatitis because of the defatting action of acetone, but the slow absorption through the skin does not appear to be of toxicologic significance. Eyes contaminated with acetone may have transient, moderate irritation and can be expected to heal completely.

Treatment: Ingestion—if a large amount is ingested, induce emesis (Ipecac Syrup, p. 3) or perform gastric lavage (p. 4). Inhalation—remove the patient from the exposure. Prevent hypoxia by use of intubation, respiratory support, and oxygen as needed. Eyes—flush the eyes thoroughly (p. 6).

There is no way to speed up elimination. Use symptomatic and supportive therapy.

Laboratory: Serum acetone, blood sugar, and urine acetone are useful to monitor the severity of ingestion or inhalation.

References:

Strong, G.F.: Acute acetone poisoning. Canad. Med. Assn. J., 51:359, 1944.
Gitelson, W., Werczberger, A., and Herman, J.B.: Coma and hyperglycemia following drinking of acetone. Diabetes, 15:810, 1966.
Harris, L.C., and Jackson, R.H.: Acute acetone poisoning caused by setting fluid for immobilizing casts. Brit. Med. J., 2:1024, 1952.
Haggard, H.W., Greenberg, L.A., and Turner, J.M.: The physiological principles governing the action of acetone together with determination of toxicity. J. Indust. Hyg. Toxicol., 26:133, 1944.

Adhesive Cements and Glues

Type of Product: Adhesives containing aromatic hydrocarbon solvents.

Ingredients/Description: Toluene and xylene are aromatic hydrocarbons used widely as solvents for rubber and plastic cements. Benzene, which was used in the past, and other organic substances may be contaminants.

Toxicity: Toluene and xylene may cause local irritation on the skin or if swallowed. Inhalation (intentional abuse or accidental) causes central nervous system excitation then depresssion. Renal tubular acidosis and hepatic injury have been reported after exposure to toluene. Chronic inhalation abuse has been inconstantly associated with evidence of renal damage, hepatic injury, peripheral neuropathy, and chronic encephalopathy. Sudden death has occurred, probably because of sensitization of the myocardium to epinephrine and subsequent ventricular fibrillation; respiratory arrest more frequently has been reported as the cause. Toluene and xylene have no known bone marrow toxicity.

Benzene causes depression of the central nervous system and has been associated with bone marrow depression; 15 ml of benzene has been reported to be lethal in man.

Symptoms and Findings: Inhalation or ingestion causes a burning sensation in the throat, nausea, vomiting, dizziness, headache, weakness, euphoria, tremors, shallow respiration, ventricular arrhythmias, paralysis, convulsions, and coma. Dermatitis occurs with chronic skin exposure. Aplastic anemia may result from benzene poisoning, and leukemia may develop after a delay of 20 years or more.

Treatment: If more than a small amount of the adhesive (10 ml) is ingested, induce emesis (Ipecac Syrup, p. 3) or perform gastric lavage (p. 4). If the product is inhaled, remove the patient from the exposure, prevent hypoxia by use of intubation, respiratory support, and oxygen as needed. Monitor for cardiac arrhythmias.

If the product is aspirated, observe the patient and treat as for chemical pneumonitis.

There is no way to speed up elimination. Use symptomatic and supportive care.

References:

Bass, M.: Sudden sniffing death. J.A.M.A., **212**:2075, 1970.

Alpert, J.J., and Lovejoy, F.H., Jr.: Management of acute childhood poisoning. Curent Problems in Pediatrics, Vol. 1, No. 5, March 1971.

Taher, S.M., Anderson, R.J., McCartney, R., Popovtzer, M., and Schrier, R.W.: Renal tubular acidosis associated with the toluene "sniffing." New Engl. J. Med., **290**:765, 1974.

Knox, J.W., and Nelson, J.R.: Permanent encephalopathy from toluene inhalation. New Engl. J. Med., **275**:1494, 1966.

Hayden, J.W., Peterson, R.G., and Bruckner, J.V.: Toxicology of toluene (Methylbenzene): Review of current literature. Clin. Toxicol., **11**:549, 1977.

Haley, T.J.: Evaluation of the health effects of benzene inhalation. Clin. Toxicol., **11**:531, 1977.

Two other classifications of adhesives are commonly encountered in the 1980's and deserve consideration.

Epoxy Resins and Polyamines

Ingredients/Description: The resins are usually long-chain polymers. Viscosity varies from liquids to solids, and solvents added may be glycidyl ether, styrene oxide, or styrene epoxide. Cold curing agents usually involve polyamines. Fumes of both the resin and curing agent are emitted during the curing process.

Toxicity: The epoxy resins may cause skin irritation and/or sensitization. Polyamine hardeners are alkaline caustic on inhalation and contact.

Symptoms and Findings: Epoxy resin may produce burns to the skin, dermatitis, lacrimation, or sneezing. Ingestion of large amounts may cause central nervous system depression.

Polyamines may cause severe burns of the skin and mucous membranes on contact. Inhalation may produce severe irritation of the respiratory tract.

Fumes of cured epoxy resins may cause pruritis, periorbital edema, conjunctivitis, coughing, asthmatic attacks, and bronchospasm.

Treatment: Prevent hypoxia by use of intubation, respiratory support, and oxygen as needed. Observe for the development of respiratory tract irritation, bronchitis, or pneumonia. In ingestion, **do not** induce emesis. If the patient is able to swallow competently (p. 5), offer one-half to one glass of water or milk. Obtain consultation with an endoscopist. Treat as an alkaline caustic (see Alkali, p. 30).

If on the skin, immediately decontaminate copiously with soap and water (p. 6). If irritation or pain persist, burn treatment may be needed.

If the eyes are contaminated, irrigate them for 15 minutes (p. 6). An ophthalmic examination should then be performed.

Cyanoacrylates (Super Glue, Krazy Glue)

Ingredients/Description: Available in small tubes under a variety of trade names.

Toxicity: The main effect is rapid adhesion between any surfaces. The adhesive action occurs rapidly on exposure to air, pressure, or slight moisture. Ingestion does not cause systemic toxicity, but it may cause adhesion on mucous membrane surfaces.

If heated and inhaled, these substances may cause eye and respiratory tract irritation. Cyanide is not released.

Symptoms and Findings: On the skin, there may be limited irritation in the area of adhesion.

In the mouth, a grayish white plaque may be evident where the substance is adhered.

When in the eye, the eyelids may be sealed together. The conjunctival areas may show irritation, and the cornea may become cloudy.

Treatment: Contaminated eyes should be irrigated, if possible, with an isotonic solution (p. 6) for 15 minutes. Do not pull the eyelids apart. If irritation and pain persist, obtain an ophthalmologic consultation. Even when clouding of the cornea occurs, no significant, permanent damage is anticipated.

If in the mouth, leave the substance alone to wear off. The same applies to the skin near the mucous membranes.

Soaking skin areas for several hours with acetone (not near the eye or mucous membranes), warm water, or mineral or vegetable oil may soften the bond sufficiently to separate the tissue surfaces.

References:

Grant, W.M.: Toxicology of the Eye, ed. 2. Springfield, Illinois: Charles C Thomas, pp. 338-339, 1974.

First Aid Sheet: Information on First Aid and Casualty – On Treatment for Adhesion of Human Skin to Itself If Caused by Cyanoacrylate Adhesives. Loctite Corporation, Newington, Connecticut, 1977.

deFonseka, C.P.: Danger of instant adhesives. Brit. Med. J., 2:1447, December 11, 1976.

Arena, J.M.: Poisoning – Toxicology, Symptoms, Treatments, ed. 3. Springfield, Illinois: Charles C Thomas, p. 569, 1974.

Deichman, W.B., and Gerarde, H.W.: Toxicology of Drugs and Chemicals. New York: Academic Press, pp. 241-242, 1969.

Fawcett, I.W., Taylor, A.J., and Pepys, J.: Asthma due to inhaled chemical agents: Epoxy resin systems containing phthalic acid anhydride, trimellitic acid anhydride and triethylene tetramine. Clin. Allerg., 7:1, 1977.

Hamilton, A., and Hardy, H.L.: Industrial Toxicology, ed. 3, revised. Acton, Massachusetts: Publishing Sciences Group, pp. 332-333, 1974.

Krajewska, D., and Rudzki, E.: Sensitivity to epoxy resins and triethylenetetramine. Contact Dermatitis, 2:135, 1976.

Sargent, E.V., Mitchell, C.A., and Brubaker, R.E.: Respiratory effects of occupational exposure to an epoxy resin system. Arch. Environ. Health, 31:236, 1976.

Alkali

Type of Product: Alkali is an ingredient in oven cleaners, drain cleaners, electric dishwasher detergent, Clinitest tablets, lye, lime, some laundry detergents, hair straighteners, etc.

Ingredients/Description: Examples of alkalis are sodium hydroxide, potassium hydroxide, trisodium phosphate, wood ash lye, sodium or potassium carbonate, calcium oxide. Pure or concentrated products occur as liquid, powder, crystals, or compressed beads.

Toxicity: The caustic action of all compounds depends on the concentration of free base at the mucosal, conjunctival, or skin surface. Therefore, the size of the dose is not the only determinant of toxicity. A small amount, such as one crystal of alkaline drain cleaner, can produce serious burns. More than 2 to 4% sodium hydroxide has the potential of causing injury. Solid alkali may adhere to the oral mucosa and produce esophageal damage; gastric damage may occur when large quantities are ingested. Concentrated liquid alkali produces mouth, esophageal, and gastric injury of a more severe nature in almost all patients.

The absence of oral burns does not exclude esophageal damage, and oral burns do not always indicate esophageal damage.

Symptoms and Findings: There may be skin burns, eye burns, oral burns (these burns may appear white), or burning pain in the mouth, throat, and stomach; drooling and dysphagia; vomitus containing mucous and later containing blood. Shock may develop. Death may be the result of shock or asphyxia, sometimes caused by glottic edema. In 2 to 4 days after apparent improvement, sudden pain in the abdomen or chest and shock may develop, indicating perforation of the stomach or esophagus. Esophageal stricture may develop as a complication 2 to 3 weeks after ingestion.

Treatment: A burn occurs when there is contact of tissue and a strong alkali. There is no antidote, but attempts can be made to prevent further damage. Do not induce emesis or perform gastric lavage. If the patient is able to swallow competently (see p. 5), dilute the ingested alkali immediately with one-half to one glass of water or milk, then give nothing by mouth. Do not attempt to neutralize the ingested alkali with vinegar or citrus juice. Tracheostomy may be indicated for obstruction from laryngeal edema. Maintain circulation (fluids, plasma, drugs). Obtain a consultation with an endoscopist within the first few hours. Any symptomatic patient should receive steroids while awaiting esophagoscopy (prednisone, 2 mg/kg per day). The use of broad spectrum anti-biotics is not uniformly accepted. If steroids and antibiotics are used, they can be discontinued if esophagoscopy does not reveal burns.

The timing of esophagoscopy for determining the extent of corrosive damage varies. Some believe it should be done between 12 and 24 hours after ingestion. Others believe a delay of 48 to 72 hours may allow the edema to subside so a more thorough examination is possible. Later, however, examinations must be done with increased caution to avoid perforation. Barium swallow in the acute stage does not yield adequate information and does not take the place of esopha-goscopy. A barium swallow in 7 to 10 days can confirm the absence of a burn. The degree of stricture formation may be followed with serial esophagograms.

For external burns, strip off saturated clothing, brush off any alkali particles, and flush the burned areas with large volumes of water.

If alkali gets into the eyes, irrigate them for at least 30 minutes (see p. 6). The patient must be seen by an ophthal-mologist.

References:

Ashcraft, K.W., and Simon, J.L.: Accidental caustic ingestion in childhood: A review. Pathogenesis and current concepts of treat-ment. Texas Med., 68:86, 1972.

Haller, J.A., Jr., Andrews, H.G., White, J.J., Tamer, M.A., and Cleve-land, W.W.: Pathophysiology and management of acute corrosive burns of the esophagus: Results of treatment in 285 children. J. Pediat. Surg., 6:578, 1971.

Johnson, E.E.: A study of corrosive esophagitis. Laryngoscope, 73:1651, 1963.

Leape, L.L., Ashcraft, K.W., Scarpelli, D.G., and Holder, T.M.: Hazard to health – Liquid lye. New Engl. J. Med., 284:578, 1971.

The management of lye burns of the esophagus. The Medical Letter, Vol. 14, No. 6, p. 18, 1972.

Grant, W.M.: Toxicology of the Eye, ed. 2. Springfield, Illinois: Charles C Thomas, pp. 96-101, 1974.

Smith, R.E., and Conway, B.: Alkali retinopathy. Arch. Ophthalmol., 94:81, 1976.

Hawkins, D.B., Demeter, M.J., and Barnett, T.E.: Caustic ingestion: Controversies in management. A review of 214 cases. Laryn-goscope, 90:98, 1980.

Stannard, M.W.: Corrosive esophagitis in children: Assessment by esophagogram. Amer. J. Dis. Child., 132:596, 1978.

Knopp, R.: Caustic ingestions. J. Amer. Coll. Emerg. Phys., 8:329, 1979.

Ammonia

Type of Product: Household cleaner, ammonia ampules, Ammonia Spirits.

Ingredients/Description: So-called household ammonia contains 7% ammonia. Preparations for commercial use may contain up to 30% ammonia.

Toxicity: Depending on the concentration of ammonia, burns of the mouth, throat, and esophagus may occur. Eye and skin irritations and/or burns may also occur. General cleaning formulations with ammonia seldom produce burns, whereas full strength ammonia may. The more concentrated the product, the more caustic it is.

When mixed with sodium hypochlorite (bleach), chloramine gas is liberated, and pulmonary symptoms similar to those produced by chlorine gas may occur.

Symptoms and Findings: Eye contact with liquid or vapor may lead to conjunctivitis, corneal irritation, and, depending on its strength, possible permanent damage.

Inhalation may lead to laryngeal edema, stridor, bronchorrhea, or cyanosis. Absorption of ammonia has been associated with convulsions and coma.

Treatment: Do not induce emesis. If the patient is able to swallow, dilute the ingested substance with one-half to one glass of water or milk. Do not attempt to neutralize the ingested product with vinegar or citrus juice. Consultation with an endoscopist is necessary if the patient ingested a substance containing 20% or more ammonia, has pain, or is drooling.

If the substance is spilled on the skin, remove saturated clothing and flush the skin with water (p. 6).

If there is eye exposure, flush the eye with copious amounts of water (p. 6) and consider an examination by an ophthalmologist.

References:

Caplin, M.: Ammonia gas poisoning: Forty-seven cases in a London shelter. Lancet, 2:95, 1941.

Norton, R.A.: Esophageal and antral strictures due to ingestion of household ammonia: Report of two cases. New Engl. J. Med., 262:10, 1960.

Dunn, S., and Ozere, R.L.: Ammonia inhalation poisoning – household variety. Canad. Med. Assn. J., 94:401, 1966.

Faigel, H.C.: Mixtures of household cleaning agents. New Engl. J. Med., 271:618, 1964.

Amphetamine

Type of Product: Central nervous system stimulant, sympathomimetic agent, diet pills.

Manufacturer: Refer to the specific drug in the *Physicians' Desk Reference.* Also there are a wide variety of illegal analogs.

Ingredients/Description: The drugs include amphetamine sulfate (Benzedrine), dextroamphetamine sulfate (Dexampex, Dexedrine, Ferndex, Oxydess II, Spancap No. 1), methamphetamine hydrochloride (Desoxyn, Methampex), amphetamine mixtures of various amphetamine salts and dextroamphetamine (Amphaplex, Obetrol, Delcobese), dextroamphetamine and prochlorperazine (Eskatrol), amphetamine-dextroamphetamine resin (Biphetamine) and other sympathomimetic amines such as phentermine hydrochloride (Phentrol, Tora, Adipex, Delcophen, Fastin, Obephen, Unifast, Wilpowr, Ionamin, Parmine), chlorphentermine hydrochloride (Presate), clortermine hydrochloride (Voranil), phenmetrazine hydrochloride (Preludin) phendimetrazinetartrate (Adphen, Anorex, Aptrol, Bacarate, Bontil PDM, Di-ap-trol, Dietabs, Ex-obese, Limit, Melfiat, Metra, Obalan, Obepar, Obestrol, Obeval, Obezine, Omnibese, PDM, PE-DE-EM, Phenazine, Phendimead, Phenzine, Plegine, Reton, Sprx, Statobex, Stim, Trimstat, Trimtabs, Weightrol, Weh-less, Prelu), benzphetamine hydrochloride (Didrex), diethylpropion (Depletite, Tenuate, Tepanil), mazindol (Sanorex), fenfluramine hydrochloride (Pondimin).

Check the *Physicians' Desk Reference* or *Facts and Comparisons* for specific drug concentrations.

Amphetamines frequently are encountered in drug abuse situations and are called by a variety of "street" names such as: Speed, Tips, Bennies, A's, Footballs, Pep Pills, Crossroads, Purple Hearts, Co-pilots, and Wakeups. "Speed freaks" are intravenous amphetamine users.

Toxicity: A lethal dose can be as little as 5 mg/kg for a child and 20 mg/kg for an adult. There is considerable individual variation in the response to these drugs, and there are indications children are more susceptible to toxicity than adults. Amphetamine in doses of 30 mg (by history) has caused severe reactions, yet some patients have survived after doses of 400 to 500 mg. Death in adults has resulted from as little as 120 mg ingested amphetamine. Large doses can be tolerated after chronic use of the drug. These drugs are frequently combined with a barbiturate, and the patient should be treated accordingly.

Symptoms and Findings: Nausea, vomiting, dry mouth with foul odor, dilated pupils, hallucinations, psychosis with peculiar repetitive mannerisms of the extremities or mouth or jaw, delirium, spasms, convulsions, and coma can occur. Lassitude, restlessness, dizziness, tremor, hyperreflexia, talkativeness, tenseness, irritability, hyperpyrexia, and insomnia may also occur. Cardiovascular effects include headache, chilliness, sweating, pallor, flushing, palpitation, cardiac arrhythmias, angina, hypertension or hypotension, and circulatory collapse. External stimuli may increase the state of hyperactivity in acute intoxication. The presence of sweating differentiates this from an atropine ingestion.

Limited information suggests newborn infants of amphetamine-using mothers may show withdrawal symptoms of dysphoria, significant lassitude, or agitation.

Treatment: Induce emesis (Ipecac Syrup, p. 3) or perform gastric lavage (p. 4). Give activated charcoal (p. 4), followed by saline laxative (p. 5). Minimize external stimuli. Sedation may be beneficial; however, it is difficult to achieve with safety and may aggravate postexcitatory depression. Chlorpromazine (Thorazine) has been shown to be beneficial in the treatment of central nervous system effects of an overdose of licit amphetamine. The initial recommended dose should not exceed 1.0 mg/kg, intramuscularly, as directed by the presence of excitation, convulsions, and concomitant hypertension.

When an amphetamine-barbiturate combination has been taken, a smaller dose of chlorpromazine, not exceeding 0.5 mg/kg, must be used to minimize the postexcitatory depression from the barbiturate.

In illicit amphetamine-like drugs, such as STP, DMT, and

MDA, chlorpromazine should **not** be used because severe hypotension may occur.

Chlorpromazine should not be used to treat toxicity from chronic amphetamine abuse.

Haloperidol and droperidol have been reported as effective antagonists of the central stimulatory effects of amphetamines.

Patients who become hyperthermic may need to be cooled. Repeated doses of activated charcoal may be advisable. Limited clinical documentation indicates forced acid diuresis may somewhat increase excretion of the amphetamine and its metabolites. Peritoneal dialysis has been used successfully.

References:

Baldessarini, R.J.: Symposium: Behavior modification by drugs. I. Pharmacology of the amphetamines. Pediatrics, **49**:694, 1972.

Espelin, D.E., and Done, A.K.: Amphetamine poisoning. Effectiveness of chlorpromazine. New Engl. J. Med., **278**:1361, 1968.

Gary, N.E., and Saidi, P.: Methamphetamine intoxication: A speedy new treatment. Amer. J. Med., **64**:537, 1978.

Ginsberg, M.D., Hertzman, M., and Schmidt-Nowara, W.W.: Amphetamine intoxication with coagulopathy, hyperthermia, and reversible renal failure. A syndrome resembling heatstroke. Ann. Intern. Med., **73**:81, 1970.

Wallace, H.E., Neumayer, F., and Gutch, C.F.: Amphetamine poisoning and peritoneal dialysis: A case report. Amer. J. Dis. Child., **108**:657, 1964.

Wan, S.H., Matin, S.B., and Azarnoff, D.L.: Kinetics, salivary excretion of amphetamine isomers, and effect of urinary pH. Clin. Pharmacol. Ther., **23**:585, 1978.

Eriksson, M., Larsson, G., Winbladh, B., and Zetterstrom, R.: The influence of amphetamine addiction on pregnancy and the newborn infant. Acta Paediat. Scand., **67**:95, 1978.

Arsenic

Type of Product: Pesticide.

Ingredients/Description: Arsenic is available as trivalent, pentavalent, and organic compounds.

Toxicity: See Table 6. Humans are more sensitive than rodents to arsenic. Acute poisoning usually is associated with accidental ingestion of arsenic-containing pesticides.

Symptoms and Findings: There may be gastroenteritis; burning pains in the esophagus and stomach; vomiting; watery or bloody diarrhea; dehydration with thirst and muscular cramps; occasional convulsions; stupor; cold, clammy skin; or coma. Electrocardiogram changes and renal failure may occur. Some arsenicals are radiopaque and may be seen on x-ray of the abdomen. Death may result from circulatory failure or acute respiratory failure. If chronic overexposure is suspected, check for diarrhea, hyperpigmentation, hyperkeratosis, circumscribed edema (lower eyelids and ankles), Mee's lines, garlic breath, excessive salivation and sweating, mental changes, polyneuritis, bone marrow abnormalities, and electrocardiogram changes. Neurologic manifestations, if present, may be refractory to treatment but improve in time.

Treatment: Induce emesis (Ipecac Syrup, p. 3) or perform gastric lavage (p. 4), followed by a demulcent. In the relatively asymptomatic patient, blood arsenic and 24-hour urine arsenic levels may be determined (use the same containers as for lead determinations). Specific treatment may be needed. Give acutely ill patients intravenous fluids to correct dehydration and electrolyte deficiencies. Treat shock

Table 6
Comparative Acute Toxicities of Some Common Arsenicals*

Arsenical	Oral LD_{50} in Rats (mg/kg)	Estimated Mortality in Human Poisoning
Arsenic trioxide	385	12%
Sodium arsenite	42	65%
Calcium arsenite	ca. 275	?
Lead arsenite	1,500+	5%
Ortho crabgrass killer†	3,719	none known

*From Done, A. K.: . . . And old lace. Emerg. Med., 5:246, January, 1973.

†Produce containing 8% each of only mildly toxic octyl NH_4 and dodecyl NH_4 methanearsonate.

with oxygen, blood, and fluids as needed. Monitor electro-cardiograms and renal function. Institute chelation therapy immediately.

BAL (dimercaprol) is an effective chelating agent for arsenic. Give BAL, by deep intramuscular injection, 2 to 4 mg/kg per dose every 4 hours. The dose may be tapered after 48 hours, depending on the condition of the patient and the amount of arsenic in the urine.

d-Penicillamine may be used to chelate arsenic in milder cases or for prolonged therapy following an acute episode; 100 mg/kg to a maximum dose of 1 gm per day in four divided doses may be given orally on an empty stomach (no food 1 hour before to 1 hour after the dose). Monitor arsenic concentration in 24-hour urine specimen (use the same container as for lead). Therapy should continue until the urine arsenic is less than 50 µg/l.

Hemodialysis is effective in reducing blood arsenic levels in acute poisoning. Chelation therapy should proceed at the same time. Renal failure may be transient.

Laboratory: In young children, little arsenic is expected to be found in the blood from environmental sources. In adults, 3 to 7 µg/100 ml blood is considered the normal range.

A 24-hour urine specimen is considered by many a better index for diagnosis. Fifty micrograms per liter and over is indicative of excessive exposure. (Ingestion of shellfish may give a temporary elevation.)

References:

Chisolm, J.J., Jr.: Poisoning due to heavy metal. Pediat. Clin. N. Amer., **17**:591, 1970.

Peterson, R.G., and Rumack, B.H.: d-Penicillamine therapy of acute arsenical poisoning. J. Pediat., **91**:661, 1977.

Giberson, A., Vazir, N.D., Mirahamadi, K., and Rosen, S.M.: Hemodialysis of acute arsenic intoxication with transient renal failure. Arch. Intern. Med., **136**:1303, 1976.

Chhuttani, P.N., Chawla, L.S., and Sharma, T.D.: Arsenical neuro-pathy. Neurology, **17**:269, 1967.

Goldsmith, S., and From, A.H.L.: Arsenic-induced atypical ventricular tachycardia. New Engl. J. Med., **303**:1096, 1980; and Atypical ventricular tachycardia after arsenic poisoning (Letters), **304**:607, 1981.

Kyle, R.A., and Pease, G.L.: Hematologic aspects of arsenic intoxication. New Engl. J. Med., **273**:18, 1965.

Westhoff, D.D., Samaha, R.J., and Barnes, A., Jr.: Arsenic intoxication as a cause of megaloblastic anemia. Blood, 45:241, 1975.

Atropine

Type of Product: Anticholinergic agent, belladonna alkaloid.

Ingredients/Description: An ingredient in many gastrointestinal and ophthalmic preparations. Proprietary sleep aids, asthma powders, plants such as jimson weed, Angel's trumpet, henbane, and deadly nightshade contain related alkaloids, such as scopolamine.

Toxicity: There will be a rapid onset of symptoms, which may persist for 48 hours or longer. As little as 10 mg has been fatal in a child. Intoxication in young children has been reported from administration of eye drops. There is considerable individual variation in response to these drugs, and there are indications children are more susceptible to toxicity than adults.

Symptoms and Findings: The patient may have dilated pupils, blurred vision, and photophobia; dry, burning sensation of the mouth; excessive thirst; difficulty in swallowing and talking; hyperthermia; generalized flushing (an erythematous rash may appear; this is more common in children); hot, dry skin; headache; nausea; excitement; confusion; delirium; convulsions; rapid pulse (may not be prominent in infants; palpitations in adults); rapid respirations; and urinary urgency with difficulty in micturition. Abdominal distension is possible in infants. Large amounts of atropine may cause paralysis, coma, and circulatory collapse. Death results from respiratory failure.

Treatment: If atropine is ingested, induce emesis (Ipecac Syrup, p. 3) or perform gastric lavage (p. 4). The motility of the gastrointestinal tract will be considerably reduced by belladonna alkaloids and anticholinergic agents, so there may be considerable retrieval hours later. Decontaminate the lower gastrointestinal tract (p. 5). Support respiration.

Physostigmine, which may be used for a diagnostic trial, rapidly reverses symptoms of anticholinergic poisoning.

Convulsions, hyperthermia, severe tachycardia, and/or arrhythmias and hypertension are all indications for the therapeutic use of physostigmine. Hallucinations may also be an indication if the patient may harm himself or others. Be aware that physostigmine is rapidly destroyed, and the patient's symptoms may return within 1 to 2 hours. For the physostigmine dose in children: start with 0.5 mg, slowly intravenously, over 1 minute. Repeat this dose at 5- to 10-minute intervals up to 2 mg or until reversal of the toxic effects. In adults, start with 1 mg, slowly intravenously, over 1 to 3 minutes. The dose may be repeated at 5- to 10-minute intervals up to 4 mg or until reversal of the toxic effects. The lowest effective dose should be repeated if life-threatening signs recur.

Neostigmine is ineffective in reversing the effects of atropine on the central nervous system.

If hyperthermia occurs, use tepid water sponging along with physostigmine. Monitor for urinary retention, and catheterize the patient if necessary.

Phenothiazines potentiate the anticholinergic effects of the belladonna alkaloids and should not be used.

References:

Mackenzie, A.L., and Pigott, J.F.G.: Atropine overdose in three children. Brit. J. Anesth., 43:1088, 1971.

Baker, J.P., and Farley, J.D.: Toxic psychosis following atropine eyedrops. Brit. Med. J., 2:1390, 1958.

Gosseslin, R.E., Hodge, H.C., Smith, R.R., and Gleason, M.N.: Clinical Toxicology of Commercial Products: Acute Poisoning, ed. 4. Baltimore: Williams and Wilkins, Section III, pp. 43-46, 1976, reprinted 1977.

Mikolich, J.R., Paulson, G.W., and Cross, C.J.: Acute anticholinergic syndrome due to Jimson seed ingestion: Clinical and laboratory observation in six cases. Ann. Intern. Med., 83:321, 1975.

Rumack, B.H.: Anticholinergic poisoning: Treatment with physostigmine. Pediatrics, 52:449, 1973.

Goodman, A.G., Gilman, L.S., and Gilman, A.: The Pharmacological Basis of Therapeutics, ed. 6. New York: Macmillan Publishing Company, Inc., 1980.

Barbiturates

Type of Product: Sedatives, hypnotics, and anticonvulsants.

Manufacturer: Refer to specific drug in *Physicians' Desk Reference.*

Ingredients/Description: For convenience, barbiturates may be classified as to their duration of action as ultra short, short, intermediate, or long acting. Examples are given in Table 7. Barbiturates are in tablet, capsule, and liquid forms.
   Primidone is partially (15%) metabolized to phenobarbital.

Toxicity: Barbiturates are readily absorbed after ingestion. They become reversibly bound to serum albumin to various extents. Most barbiturates are metabolized chiefly, but not solely, in the liver. Short-acting barbiturates are rapidly degraded by the liver, and only negligible quantities are excreted unchanged in the urine. Overdose may cause deep and rapid onset of coma and severe complications. Long-acting barbiturates are slowly metabolized by the liver, and about 25% of a dose is excreted unchanged in the urine.
   Concomitant alcohol, antihistamine, or tranquilizer ingestions may cause deeper coma than anticipated for the serum barbiturate level. Addicts and seizure patients on medication routinely may exhibit a higher tolerance. Metabolic elimination is more rapid in young patients than in the elderly or infants.
   The generally recommended hypnotic dose for children of

Table 7
Barbiturates

Long Acting	Intermediate Acting	Short Acting	Ultra-short Acting
Barbital (Veronal) Phenobarbital (Luminal) Mephobarbital (Mebaral)	Pentobarbital (Nembutal) Amobarbital (Amytal) Butabarbital (Butisol) Vinbarbital (Delvinal) Probarbital (Ipral)	Secobarbital (Seconal) Allybarbituric acid	Thiopental (Pentothal) Thiamytal (Surital)

Table 8
Actions of Barbiturates

Action	Long Acting	Intermediate Acting	Short Acting	Extra-short Acting
Therapeutic dose				
Action Peak	6 hr	3-6 hr	3 hr	seconds
Onset	1 hr	1 hr	minutes	seconds
Dose duration	10-12 hr	6-8 hr	4-8 hr	minutes
Potential toxic dose	65-75 mg/kg	40-50 mg/kg	40-50 mg/kg	
Potential fatal dose	Barbital 10 gm Phenobarbital 6-10 mg	2-3 gm	Pentobarbital (2-3 gm) Secobarbital (2-3 gm)	
Liquid partition coefficient*	Barbital 1 Phenobarbital 3		Pentobarbital 39 Secobarbital 52	
Plasma protein binding (%)	Barbital 5 Phenobarbital 20		Pentobarbital 35 Secobarbital 44	
Plasma level Fatal (mg/dl)	Barbital 15 Phenobarbital 8-10	Amobarbital 3.5 Butabarbital 3.5	Pentobarbital or Secobarbital 3.5	

Coma (mg/dl)	Phenobarbital 3-5	Amobarbital 1-3 Butabarbital 1-3	Pentobarbital or Secobarbital 1-2
pKa	Barbital 7.74 Phenobarbital 7.24	Amobarbital 7.75 Butabarbital 7.74	Pentobarbital 7.96 Secobarbital 7.90
Comment	Barbital—Diuresis increases excretion Phenobarbital— alkalinization and diuresis increase excretion 100%	Osmotic diuresis	Diuresis increases excretion <20%

*Between methyl chloride and an aqueous buffer. Higher coefficients reflect greater solubility in lipid.

phenobarbital, barbital, secobarbital, and pentobarbital is 2 to 3 mg/kg. The average toxic dose is five times the hypnotic dose. The lethal dose of barbiturate varies with many factors and cannot be stated with certainty. Severe poisoning is likely to occur when 10 times the full hypnotic dose is taken at one time (Table 8).

Withdrawal syndromes (including in the neonate) have been described and require specialized treatment management.

Symptoms and Findings: Low toxic dose – decreased sensory ability (6 mg/kg). Medium toxic dose – decreased motor ability. High toxic dose – decreased medullary activity.

Moderate intoxication resembles alcoholic inebriation. The patient is comatose in severe intoxication, and the level of reflex activity conforms in a general way to the intensity of the central depression. There is drowsiness, a transient period of confusion and excitement, ataxia, vertigo, slurred speech, headache, and paresthesias. Stupor progresses to coma; there is a progressive loss of deep reflexes and a loss of response to pain. The Babinski reflex is positive. Respiration is affected early. Breathing may be slow or rapid and shallow. Cheyne-Stokes rhythm may be present. Respiratory minute volume is diminished, and hypoxemia and respiratory acidosis may develop. There is progressive cardiovascular collapse with a weak, rapid pulse; cold, sweating skin; hypotension; and cyanosis. Respiratory complications (atelectasis, pulmonary edema, and bronchopneumonia) and renal failure frequently occur. Death is caused by respiratory arrest.

Bullous skin lesions suggest coma over 12 hours' duration. Pupils are initially small and dilate terminally.

Treatment: Prevent hypoxia by use of intubation, respiratory support, and oxygen as needed. Analeptics should not be used. Maintain blood pressure with intravenous fluids and vasopressors (dopamine or metaraminol) as needed. Empty the stomach by emesis (Ipecac Syrup, p. 3) or perform a gastric lavage (p. 4). If in a coma, protect the airway. Decontaminate the lower gastrointestinal tract (p. 5). Multiple oral doses of activated charcoal should be administered in phenobarbital overdose as it has been shown to reduce the serum half-life and increase the nonrenal clearance over 50%. Institute supportive and symptomatic care.

Forced alkaline diuresis (if not in shock) using sodium bicarbonate (3 to 5 mEq/kg, intravenously) along with furosemide or mannitol will promote excretion of phenobarbital. Osmotic diuresis is of limited value for other barbiturates.

Peritoneal or hemodialysis for long-acting barbiturate intoxication should be considered for the following indications: (1) progressive deterioration with conservative therapy, (2) prolonged coma, and (3) renal or hepatic failure with impaired excretory routes. Dialysis may be used to correct acid-base, electrolyte, and fluid disturbance in both short- and long-acting barbiturate poisoning. Charcoal hemoperfusion may be helpful in the patient who is severely intoxicated.

Bullae are treated as a second degree burn.

References:

Hadden, J., Johnson, K., Smith, S., Price, L., and Giardina, E.: Acute barbiturate intoxication. Concepts of management. J.A.M.A., 209:893, 1969.

Mann, J.B., and Sandberg, D.H.: Therapy of sedative overdosage. Pediat. Clin. N. Amer., 17:617, 1970.

Setter, J.G., Maher, J.F., and Schreiner, G.E.: Barbiturate intoxication. Evaluation of therapy including dialysis in the large series selectively referred because of severity. Arch. Intern. Med., 117:224, 1966.

Shubin, H., and Weil, M.H., Shock associated with barbiturate intoxication. J.A.M.A., 215:263. 1971.

Matthew, H.: Barbiturates. Clin. Toxicol., 8:495, 1975.

Goodman J.M., et al.: Barbiturate intoxication: Morbidity and mortality. West. J. Med., 124:179, 1976.

Desmond, M.M.. Schwanecke, R.P., Wilson, G.S., Yasunaga, S., and Burgdorff, I.: Maternal barbiturate utilization and neonatal withdrawal symptomatology. J. Pediat., 80:190, 1972.

Berg, M.J., Berlinger, W.G., Goldberg, M.J., Spector, R., and Johnson, G.F.: Acceleration of the body clearance of phenobarbital by oral activated charcoal. New Engl. J. Med., 307:642, 1982.

Benzodiazepines

Type of Product: Sedative, tranquilizer, anticonvulsant.

Ingredients/Description: Benzodiazepine is found in the products given in the following list as well as in a variety of other products.

Diazepam (Valium)	2, 5, and 10 mg tablets; 2 and 10 ml ampules (5 mg/ml)
Chlordiazepoxide (Librium)	5, 10, 25 mg capsules or tablets; 100 mg ampules
Flurazepam (Dalmane)	15 and 30 mg capsules
Oxazepam (Serax)	10, 15, 30 mg capsules; 15 mg tablets
Prazepam (Vershaw)	10 mg tablets
Clorazepate (Tranxene)	3.75, 7.5, 15 mg capsules; 11.25 and 22.5 mg sustained-release tablets
(Azene)	3.25, 6.5, and 13 mg capsules
Lorazepam (Ativan)	1 and 2 mg tablets
Chlonazepam (Clonopin)	0.5, 1, and 2 mg tablets
Halazepam (Paxipam)	20 mg tablets
Alprazolam (Xanax)	0.25, 0.5, and 1 mg tablets

Toxicity: These drugs have low toxic potential when used orally. More than 500 mg have been ingested without respiratory depression. Onset of action is rapid, with peak sedation in 1 to 2 hours. The duration of action varies with the circumstances. A great danger of all benzodiazepines is the additive effect with sedatives such as alcohol and barbiturates or other psychopharmacologic agents. Although too rapid intravenous administration of diazepam has caused apnea, few fatalities caused by benzodiazepines alone have been documented. Withdrawal syndromes (including in the neonate) have been described and require specialized management.

Symptoms and Findings: Sedation and light coma occur, but deep coma leading to respiratory depression suggests the presence of other drugs. Anticholinergic signs may occur.

Treatment: Induce emesis (Ipecac Syrup, p. 3) or perform gastric lavage (p. 4). Decontaminate the lower gastrointestinal tract (p. 5). Dialysis and forced diuresis are of no value. Prevent hypoxia by use of intubation, respiratory support, and oxygen as needed. Maintain blood pressure with intravenous fluids and vasopressors (dopamine or metaraminol) as needed.

References:

Greenblatt, D.J., Woo, E., Allen, M.D., Orsulak, P.J., and Shader, R.I.: Rapid recovery from massive diazepam overdose. J.A.M.A., 240:1872, 1978.
Welch, T.R., Rumack, B.H., and Hammond, K.: Clonazepam overdose resulting in cyclic coma. Clin. Toxicol., 10:433, 1977.
Finkle, B.S., McClaskey, K.L., and Goodman, L.S.: Diazepam and drug-associated deaths. J.A.M.A., 242:429, 1979.
Preskoin, S.H., and Denner, W.: Benzodiazepines and withdrawal psychosis. J.A.M.A., 237:36, 1977.

Bleach

Type of Product: Household liquid chlorine bleach and household liquid chlorine mildew remover.

Ingredients/Description: Household liquid chlorine bleaches usually contain between 4 and 6% sodium hypochlorite, with small amounts of other chemicals depending on the brand. In contrast, commercial liquid chlorine bleaches may be more highly concentrated. Household liquid chlorine mildew remover may have up to 5% calcium hypochlorite, making it twice as potent as household liquid chlorine bleach.

Toxicity: At one time, it was customary to classify liquid chlorine bleach with caustic alkalies; but animal experimentation and human experience after ingestion of household liquid chlorine bleaches has not substantiated this classification. However, there are reports of a few cases of ulcerative esophagitis and rare cases of esophageal stricture associated with ingestion of household bleaches. Commercial bleaches and household liquid chlorine mildew removers may be more highly concentrated and should be considered as potential alkali ingestions.

Symptoms and Findings: Ingestion—There may be a burning sensation and irritation of mucous membranes, frequently with prompt emesis. Inhalation—Gases produced by mixing chlorine bleach with strongly acidic products such as toilet bowl cleaners and rust removers (chlorine gas) or with household ammonia (chloramine gas) are irritating to mucous membranes, eyes, and the upper respiratory tract. Cough and other symptoms may indicate significant exposure (see Chlorine Gas, p. 53).

Treatment: Ingestation — Dilute the ingested product at once with water or milk (p. 5). Avoid acids. Give demulcents. Treatment is otherwise symptomatic and supportive. Esophagoscopy is not recommended unless unusually large amounts have been ingested, the patient is symptomatic, or the product was stronger than the average household bleach. Inhalation — Treatment is symptomatic and supportive. Observe the patient for pulmonary edema (see Chlorine Gas, p. 53).

References:

Pike, D.G., Peabody, J.W., Jr., Davis, E.W., and Lyons, W.S.: A reevaluation of the dangers of Clorox ingestion. J. Pediat., 63:303, 1963.

French, R.J., Tabb, H.G., and Rutledge, L.J.: Esophageal stenosis produced by ingestion of bleach: Report of 2 cases. South. Med. J., 63:1140, 1970.

Gosselin, R.E., Hodge, H.C., Smith, R.P., and Gleason, M.N.: Clinical Toxicology of Commercial Products, ed. 4. Baltimore: Williams and Wilkins Co., Section III, pp. 174-176, 1976, reprinted 1977.

Camphor

Type of Product: Topical skin medication.

Ingredients/Description:
Camphorated oil contains 20% camphor in cottonseed oil.
Campho-phenique contains 10% camphor.
Camphor spirit contains 10% camphor in alcohol.
Other products usually contain less than 5% camphor.

Toxicity: Camphor has an estimated fatal dose of 1 gm (5 ml of camphorated oil or 10 ml of Campho-phenique) when ingested by a child. The ingestion of 2 gm of camphor may produce dangerous effects in an adult, although a patient who ingested more than 40 gm of camphor recovered. Contact and inhalation exposure have been reported to cause seizures.

Symptoms and Findings: Convulsions may begin within 5 minutes after ingestion or be delayed for several hours with or without the appearance of other symptoms, which may include nausea, vomiting, a feeling of warmth, headache, confusion, vertigo, excitement, delirium, or increased muscular excitability. Coma may follow convulsions. Death may result from respiratory failure or from status epilepticus.

Treatment: Because of the possible rapid and unheralded convulsions, it is probably not advisable to induce emesis. Gastric lavage should be performed (p. 4), and the lower gastrointestinal tract should be decontaminated (p. 5). Diazepam (0.1 to 0.3 mg/kg, slowly intravenously) is useful for control of convulsions. Prevent hypoxia by use of intubation, respiratory support, and oxygen as needed. Avoid the administration of oils or alcohol, which may promote the absorption of camphor.

Provide symptomatic and supportive care. Resin hemoperfusion has been reported effective in one case.

References:

Gosselin, R.E., Hodge, H.C., Smith, R.P., and Gleason, M.N.: Clinical Toxicology of Commercial Products: Acute Poisoning, ed. 4. Baltimore: Williams and Wilkins, Section III, pp. 77-79, 1976, reprinted 1977.

Aronow, R., and Spigiel, R.W.: Implications of camphor poisoning: Therapeutic and administrative. Drug Intelligence Clin. Pharm., **10**:631, 1976.

Weiss, J., and Catalano, P.: Camphorated oil intoxication during pregnancy. Pediatrics, **52**:713, 1973.

Phelan, W.J., III: Camphor poisoning: Over-the-counter dangers. Pediatrics, **57**:428, 1976.

Kopelman, R., Mitter, S., Kelly, R., and Sunshine, I.: Camphor intoxication treated by resin hemoperfusion. J.A.M.A., **241**:727, 1979.

Skoglund, R.R., Ware, L.L., Jr., and Schanberger, J.E.: Prolonged seizures due to contact and inhalation exposure to camphor. Clin. Pediat., **16**:901, 1977.

Carbon Monoxide

Type of Product: Odorless gas emitted from incomplete combustion, and metabolic product of methylene chloride.

Source: Inadequately vented and/or malfunctioning furnaces, space heaters, gasoline motors, charcoal grills or burners, and incompetent automobile exhaust systems account for the majority of accidental exposures. Paint removal with methylene-chloride containing paint strippers results in a delayed carbon monoxide exposure. Charcoal produces great quantities of carbon monoxide, and grills brought into houses, tents, or recreation vehicles are rapidly lethal.

Toxicity: The mechanism of action is twofold: (1) Carbon monoxide binds to hemoglobin more tightly than oxygen, and the blood's oxygen-carrying capacity is reduced. Unconsciousness is caused primarily by hypoxemia. (2) Carbon monoxide poisons cellular metabolism at several enzymatic sites. For example, lesions in the globus pallidus after severe carbon monoxide poisoning are not seen with hypoxic damage and are attributed to a specific carbon monoxide mechanism.

Prediction of outcome in the comatose patient is difficult. If the patient becomes acidotic or a lesion in the globus pallidus is detected in an early CAT scan, recovery in adults may be poor or incomplete.

Symptoms and Findings: Carboxyhemoglobin levels may not correlate well with clinical findings. In acute, short exposures, carboxyhemoglobin levels between 15 and 25% are usually associated with headache (frequently the first and unrecognized symptom) and nausea. Children also may experience gastrointestinal upsets. Breathlessness occurs in some patients. Coronary pain may occur in patients with angina. At levels more than 25%, patients may suffer mental changes, including confusion, hostility, dizziness, weakness, depressed awareness of surroundings, and, ultimately, coma. There may be electrocardiographic changes. Retinal hemorrhages may be present, and delayed optic neuritis may occur. Chronic low-dose exposure may be damaging, and the patient may manifest neurologic or psychiatric dysfunction.

Treatment: Immediately establish or maintain respiration and administer 100% oxygen to all patients through the most efficient delivery device. (A mixture of oxygen with 5% carbon dioxide is no longer advised.) An unconscious or convulsing child should be intubated. If blood pressure is depressed or there is bradycardia, begin mechanical cardiac assistance without delay. Arterial blood gases and carboxyhemoglobin should be measured. **A near normal carboxyhemoglobin level does not rule out significant carbon monoxide poisoning.** The partial pressure of oxygen may be near normal, although the oxygen saturation will be reduced. The history of exposure and clinical state of the patient may dictate the therapy. Only if the blood pH is below 7.3, administer sodium bicarbonate (3 to 5 mEq/kg, intravenously, as appropriate) to correct the acidosis. Mild acidosis shifts the oxyhemoglobin disassociation curve to the right and does not need correction. If the patient is severely acidotic and remains comatose, and hyperbaric oxygen is immediately available, 1 hour at 2 to 3 ATM should be provided. If hyperbaric oxygen is not available, administer 100% oxygen at 1 ATM.

The elimination of carbon monoxide, as measured by the carboxyhemoglobin concentration, depends on 100% oxygen administration. The half-life of carbon monoxide is 5 hours in room air, but it is 1½ hours at 100% oxygen and 20 minutes with hyperbaric oxygen. Maintain the patient on oxygen to get the carboxyhemoglobin level to below 10%. Institute supportive care as needed, and monitor for complications. Myocardial damage, pulmonary edema, muscle necrosis, secondary renal involvement, ophthalmologic complications, light nerve damage, skin necrosis, cerebral edema, and various degrees of encephalopathy have all been reported.

The patient should be evaluated with regularity over several months because subtle deficiencies may not be evident immediately.

References:

Sawada, Y., Ohashi, N., Maemura, K., Yoshioka, T., Takahashi, M., Fusamoto, H., Kobayashi, H., and Sugimoto, T.: Computerized tomography as an indication of long-term outcome after acute carbon monoxide poisoning. Lancet, 1:783, 1980.

Jackson, D.L., and Menges, H.: Accidental carbon monoxide poisoning. J.A.M.A., 243:772, 1980.

Lacey, D.J.: Neurologic sequelae of acute carbon monoxide intoxication. Amer. J. Dis. Child., **135**:145, 1981.

Binder, J.W., and Roberts, R.J.: Carbon monoxide intoxication in children. Clin. Toxicol., 16:287, 1980.

Kelley, J.S., and Sophocleus, G.J.: Retinal hemorrhages in subacute carbon monoxide poisoning: Exposures in homes with blocked furnace flues. J.A.M.A., **239**:1515, 1978.

Zimmerman, S.S., and Truxal, B.: Carbon monoxide posioning. Pediatrics, **68**:215, 1981.

Cramer, C.R.: Fetal death due to accidental maternal carbon monoxide poisoning. Clin. Toxicol., 19:297, 1982.

Chloral Betaine

Type of Product: Hypnotic and sedative.

Manufacturer: Mead Johnson and Company.

Ingredients/Description: Each Beta-Chlor tablet contains chloral betaine, 870 mg (equivalent to chloral hydrate, 500 mg).

Toxicity: The central nervous system depression produced by chloral betaine in laboratory animals is approximately equivalent to that of chloral hydrate when dosage is calculated in terms of chloral hydrate content. The mean lethal dose of chloral hydrate for adults is approximately 10 gm (20 Beta-Chlor tablets). Death has occurred from as little as 4 gm. This product is detoxified in the liver and other tissues. Esophageal strictures and gastric necrosis have been reported as complications.

Symptoms and Findings: There may be gastric irritation, vomiting, hypotension, and excitement, followed by central nervous system depression, severe vasodilatation, hypothermia, slow respiration, cardiac arrhythmias, stupor, cyanosis, occasionally delirium, hypotension or pin-point pupils. The tablets are radiopaque and may be seen on x-rays of the abdomen. If the patient survives, liver and kidney damage may cause icterus and albuminuria.

Treatment: Induce emesis (Ipecac Syrup, p. 3) or perform gastric lavage (p. 4). Decontaminate the lower gastrointestinal tract (p. 5). Prevent hypoxia by use of intubation, respiratory support, and oxygen as needed. Maintain blood pressure with intravenous fluids and levarterenol as needed. Hemodialysis may be effective in severe poisoning.

References:

Nordenberg, A., Delisle, G., and Izukawa, T.: Cardiac arrhythmia in a child due to chloral hydrate ingestion. Pediatrics, 47:134, 1971.

Vaziri, N.D., Kumar, K.P. Mirahmadi, K., and Rosen, S.M.: Hemodialysis in treatment of acute chloral hydrate poisoning. South. Med. J., 70:377, 1977.

Gleich, G.J., Mongan, E.S., and Vaules, D.W.: Esophageal stricture following chloral hydrate poisoning. J.A.M.A., 201:266, 1967.

Vellar, I.D.A., Richardson, J.P., Doyle, J.C., and Keating, M.: Gastric necrosis: A rare complication of chloral hydrate intoxication. Brit. J. Surg., 59:317, 1972.

Chlorine Gas

Type of Product: Industrial gas used for manufacturing and as a disinfectant.

Ingredients/Description: Chlorine gas is a greenish-yellow gas used commercially as a disinfectant. It is liberated from household liquid chlorine bleaches, particularly in the presence of acids. When bleach is mixed with ammonia, chloramine gas is formed; and similar, though less severe, toxic effects result. Hydrochloric acid is formed if chlorine gas is mixed with water.

Toxicity: Chlorine is an active oxidizing agent with easy solubility in water and body fluids forming acid which is capable of causing rapid and extensive destruction of tissue. Depending on the severity of exposure, chlorine gas produces varying degrees of pulmonary and airway damage. It is readily detected at 3 to 5 ppm, and 1 hour of exposure may cause mild symptoms. At 15 to 30 ppm, it will cause moderate symptoms, whereas at 40 to 60 ppm the symptoms will be severe to life threatening. Exposure to 1,000 ppm (0.1%) is invariably and rapidly fatal. Low levels of chlorine (1 to 2 ppm) can usually be tolerated without undue discomfort. Some individuals may have an asthmatic response to chloramine or chlorine gas. Exposures may be classified as mild, moderate, or severe.

Symptoms and Findings: Mild – Minimal sensation of burning of mucous membranes of nose, mouth, and throat, and mild irritation of the eyes. There may be a slight cough. Moderate – Immediate, severe irritation of the mucous membranes of the nose, mouth, and throat and of the eyes is accompanied by a distresssing, sometimes paroxysmal, cough which may result in hematemesis. Headache may occur. Anxiety is usually present. A few rales may be heard in the chest; however, an x-ray of the lungs will probably be negative. Severe – Severe, productive cough; hematemesis; difficulty in breathing; and, frequently, cyanosis may be present. Vomiting may be severe. Rales may be heard throughout the lungs because of edema forming and congestion. An x-ray of the lungs may be negative, but an expirogram may show considerable expiratory reduction. Productive cough, bronchial rales, and an abnormal expirogram may persist for several days. Late – There is some evidence for chronic pulmonary effects secondary to acute chlorine exposure.

Treatment: Mild – No treatment is needed; symptoms will clear within a few minutes to an hour. Moderate – Have the patient lie down with the head and shoulders elevated. Administer oxygen in periods of a few minutes at a time until the cough and anxiety are relieved. A sedative-containing cough syrup is useful. Symptoms may abate in most patients within a few hours; however, activity should be restricted for 24 hours to observe for an exacerbation of symptoms. Severe – Have the patient rest with the head and shoulders elevated; provide warmth and reassurance. Inhalation of oxygen for periods of 15 minutes or longer is effective in alleviating symptoms and should be repeated as necessary. Sedative-containing cough syrups are indicated. Symptoms may abate; however, activity should be restricted for 24 hours to observe for an exacerbation of symptoms.

If a child has been trapped in an area of high concentration of chlorine gas, the physician is confronted with a medical emergency. Shock, coma, and respiratory arrest may be present. Treatment is supportive, and the physician must rely on clinical judgment to meet the conditions. Resuscitation measures, including inhalation of 100% oxygen and methods to combat shock, may be required. Corticosteroids may be helpful for pulmonary edema. Complications such as pneumonia should be anticipated. Intermittent positive pressure breathing with oxygen for acute pulmonary edema may be required. The use of nebulized bronchial detergent for increased mucous secretions may be helpful. For moderate and severe exposure, flush the eyes thoroughly (p. 6) and decontaminate the skin (p. 6). Obtain ophthalmologic consultation in severe exposures.

References:

Adelson, L., and Kaufman, J.: Fatal chlorine poisoning: Report of two cases with clincopathologic correlation. Amer. J. Clin. Pathol., 56:430, 1971.

Arena, J.M.: Poisoning–Toxicology, Symptoms, Treatments, ed. 3. Springfield, Illinois: Charles C Thomas, 1974.

Gay, H.H.: Exposure to chlorine gas. J.A.M.A., 183:806, 1963.

Noe, J.T.: Therapy for chlorine gas inhalation. Industrial Med. Surg., 32:411, 1963.

Chester, E.H., Kaimal, J., Payne, C.B., Jr., and Kohn, P.M.: Pulmonary injury following exposure to chlorine gas: Possible beneficial effects of steroid treatment. Chest, 72:247, 1977.

Wheater, R.H.: Hazards of exposure to chlorine gas. J.A.M.A., 230:1064, 1974.

Kaufman, J., and Burkons, D.: Clinical, roentgenologic and physiologic effects of acute chlorine exposure. Arch. Environ. Health, 23:29, 1971.

Lawson, J.J.: Chlorine exposure: A challenge to the physician. Amer. Family Physician, 23:1, 1981.

Cough and Cold Mixtures

Type of Product: Over-the-counter and prescription mixtures for the temporary relief of cough, nasal congestion, and the discomfort of colds. Some mixtures are specifically for children.

Ingredients/Description: The concentration or content of the mixtures varies with the preparation. Antihistamines are included in almost all preparations. The most common is chlorpheniramine, but methapyrilene, pyrilamine, and pheniramine are also common. A sympathomimetic drug, as an oral decongestant, is another frequent ingredient. Phenyl-propanolamine, phenylephrine, and pseudoephedrine are all commonly incorporated. Analgesics, both aspirin and aceta-minophen, are a third common ingredient. Preparations tout-ing antitussive properties may contain dextromethorphan or codeine.

Toxicity: Serious toxicity is uncommon in relation to drug use or to the number of ingestions. When toxicity occurs, it prob-ably is caused by the analgesic involved (see Salicylates or Acetaminophen) or the antihistamine. Serious toxicity from the sympathomimetic drugs is rare, although transient ele-vation of blood presssure may be observed. Dextromethor-phan may cause drowsiness or convulsions in doses in excess of 90 mg in children. Respiratory depression is rare but can occur. Codeine can cause respiratory depresssion.

Symptoms and Findings: Nausea, vomiting, headache, irrita-bility, hyperpnea, dizziness, blurred vision, dryness of the mouth, tachycardia, hypertension, arrhythmias, and palpi-tation may be present. Confusion, convulsions, and coma may ensue. Acidosis secondary to salicylates may be seen. Respiratory depression is unlikely, but it may occur secondary to dextromethorphan or codeine.

Treatment: If respiratory depression is present in patients who ingested codeine or large doses of dextromethorphan, naloxone (0.01 mg/kg, intravenously) should be given and repeated as necessary. Induce emesis (Ipecac Syrup, p. 3) or perform gastric lavage (p. 4). Decontaminate the lower gastrointestinal tract (p. 5) if a solid dosage form was ingested. If the substance contains an antihistamine and serious anticholinergic symptoms (central nevous system stimulation, convulsions, or tachycardia and/or arrhythmias) occur, consider administering physostigmine slowly intra-veously. Be aware that physostigmine is rapidly destroyed, and the patient's symptoms may return within 1 to 2 hours. For the physostigmine dose in children, start with 0.5 mg, slowly intravenously, over 1 minute. Repeat this dose at 5- to 10-minute intervals up to 2 mg or until reversal of the toxic effects. In adults, start with 1 mg, slowly intravenously, over 1 to 3 minutes. The dose may be repeated at 5- to 10-minute intervals up to 4 mg or until reversal of the toxic effects. The lowest effective dose should be repeated if life-threatening signs recur. If arrhythmias are present, consider the possibility of sympathomimetic poisoning. Propranolol (0.025 to 0.1 mg/kg, intravenously slowly over 2 to 3 minutes) may be useful, *except* in asthmatic patients where it may exacerbate bronchoconstriction. If a salicylate and/or acetaminophen is in the preparation ingested, monitor blood levels and institute appropriate therapy.

References:

Rumack, B.H., Anderson, R.J., Wolfe, R., Fletcher, E.C., and Vestal, B.K.: Ornade and anti-cholinergic toxicity: Hypertension, hallucinations, and arrhythmias. Clin. Toxicol., 7:573, 1974.

Goodman, A.G., Gilman, L.S., and Gilman, A.: The Pharmacological Basis of Therapeutics, ed. 6. New York: Macmillan Publishing Company, Inc., 1980.

Darvon Products

Type of Product: Analgesics.

Manufacturer: Eli Lilly and Company. More than 30 companies make propoxyphene.

Ingredients/Description: All products are capsules and contain the ingredients shown in Table 9. Most Darvon products contain aspirin or acetaminophen. The toxic potential of both these substances also must be considered.

Toxicity: Death has been reported in the following circumstances: not more than 1 gm in a 1-year-old child; 98 capsules (strength unspecified) in a 14-year-old girl; approximately 1.5 gm in a 19-year-old boy; approximately 650 mg in a 12-year-old child; and 1,280 mg in a 15-year-old girl. Withdrawal syndromes (including in the neonate) have been described and require specialized treatment management. Pharmacokinetic studies in humans have shown that propoxyphene is primarily eliminated by hepatic metabolism. The major metabolic pathway is demethylation to norpropoxyphene, which is, in large part, eliminated by renal excretion. Half-life is dose dependent, and there is considerable individual variation. The drug is bound to plasma proteins and is concentrated in the viscera so the level of

Table 9
Darvon Products and Other Propoxyphene-containing Preparations

Product	Color	Propoxyphene	Aspirin	Phenacetin	Caffeine	Acetaminophen
Darvon	pink cap.	32 or 65 mg	—	—	—	—
Darvon Compound	pink/gray cap.	32 mg	227 mg	162 mg	32.4 mg	—
Darvon Compound-65	red/gray cap.	65 mg	227 mg	162 mg	32.4 mg	—
Darvon with ASA	pink/red cap.	65 mg	325 mg	—	—	—
Darvon-N	buff tab.	65 mg*	—	—	—	—
Darvon-N with ASA	orange tab.	65 mg*	325 mg	—	—	—
Darvon-N (susp.)	—	32 mg/5 ml*	—	—	—	—
Darvocet-N 50	red tab.	32 mg*	—	—	—	325 mg
Darvocet-N 100	red tab.	65 mg*	—	—	—	650 mg
Dolene	pink cap.	65 mg	—	—	—	—
Dolene Compound-65	maroon/pink cap.	65 mg	227 mg	162 mg	32.4 mg	—
Dolene AP-65	pink tab.	65 mg	—	—	—	650 mg
SK-65	gray/white cap.	65 mg	—	—	—	—
SK-65 APAP	orange tab.	65 mg	—	—	—	650 mg
SK-65 Compound	burnt orange/violet cap.	65 mg	227 mg	162 mg	32.4 mg	—
Wygesic	green tab.	65 mg	—	—	—	650 mg
Generic Propoxy-phene HCl	—	32 or 65 mg	—	—	—	†

*Contains propoxyphene napsylate 50 or 100 mg, which is equivalent in propoxyphene content to 32 or 65 mg propoxyphene HCl.
†Some generic propoxyphene HCl preparations contain acetaminophen.

free drug in the blood may not reveal the severity of the overdose.

Symptoms and Findings: Nausea, vomiting, dizziness, hypotension, and central nervous system depression may be present. Severe overdoses cause respiratory depression, coma, convulsions, and respiratory and cardiac arrest.

Treatment: Unless the patient has just taken the drug and is fully alert, allowing for uncomplicated emesis (Ipecac Syrup, p. 3), the stomach should be emptied by gastric lavage (p. 4). Decontaminate the lower gastrointestinal tract (p. 5). Support respiration if breathing has stopped or its rate or depth have become too low to maintain effective ventilation. Naloxone hydrochloride (0.01 mg/kg, intravenously) is the specific antidote. The dose may be safely repeated and increased as needed if respirations are not adequate or convulsions occur (up to 20 times the recommended dose has been effectively given without complications). Establish a routine of close observation. This is important because the antidotal action of the narcotic antagonist is shorter (1 to 2 hours) than the respiratory depression from Darvon, which may last from 24 to 48 hours. Cardiac massage and intravenous epinephrine have been successful in treating cardiac arrest. Maintain blood pressure. Dialysis and charcoal hemoperfusion have not been effective. Exchange transfusion has been reported effective in two patients.

References:

Swarts, C.L.: Propoxyphene (Darvon) poisoning. A nearly fatal case with coma, convulsions, and severe respiratory depression, successfully treated with nalorphine. Amer. J. Dis. Child., 107:177, 1964.

Lovejoy, F.H., Jr., Mitchell, A.A., and Goldman, P.: The management of propoxyphene poisoning. J. Pediat., 85:98, 1974.

Tyson, H.K.: Neonatal withdrawal symptoms associated with maternal use of propoxyphene hydrochloride (Darvon). J. Pediat., 85:684, 1974.

Moore, R.A., Rumack, B.H., Conner, C.S., and Peterson, R.G.: Naloxone: Underdosage after narcotic poisoning. Amer. J. Dis. Child., 134:156, 1980.

Gram, L.F., Schou, J., Way, W.L., Heltberg, J., and Bodin, N.O.: d-Propoxyphene kinetics after single oral and intravenous doses in man. Clin. Pharm. Therap., 26:473, 1979.

Young, D.J.: Propoxyphene suicides. Arch. Intern. Med., 129:62, 1972.

Detergents

Type of Product: Detergents are synthetic, inorganic and organic products (liquids, powders, solids, or aerosols) which loosely can be divided into groups with varying degrees of toxicity: cationic, anionic, or nonionic.

Ingredients/Description: Cationic – quaternary ammonium compounds such as benzalkonium chloride (Zephiran) or hexachlorophene (pHisoHex). Anionic – alkylbenzenesulfonates (e.g., general laundry detergents such as Tide, Fab, Cheer). Nonionic – alkylaryl polyethersulfate (e.g., low-sudsing detergents and Jet Dry). Formulations of household detergents are under constant change, with many trade names remaining the same. The ingredients under a given trade name may vary from one area to another. Granular products for dishwashers have tended to be more alkaline than general household granular detergents, with various percentages of sodium tripolyphosphate, sodium metasilicate, and sodium carbonate in them.

Toxicity: Consult the regional poison control center for specific definition of the ingredients of a product. Cationic detergents are corrosive in their pure form, but corrosion is unlikely if the solution is less than 20%. The estimated fatal dose is more than 1 gm of the pure substance in an adult. These detergents appear to be inactivated by soap. Anionic and nonionic detergents and soaps are of low toxicity. However, some detergent granules and nonphosphate detergents are strongly alkaline and capable of causing corrosive lesions of the eye and mucous membranes.

Symptoms and Findings: Cationic detergents are readily absorbed from the gastrointestinal tract. Nausea, vomiting, convulsion, coma, hypotension, and shock may occur. Anionic and nonionic detergents are of low toxicity. They may cause contact dermatitis or eye irritation. Ingestion may produce mild diarrhea and vomiting. No fatalities have been reported. Detergent powders and granules may cause esophageal, gastric, respiratory tract, or eye reactions. Caustic effects may produce pharyngeal and laryngeal edema with upper airway obstruction. Esophageal burns similar to lye burns may occur. Perforation of the stomach and peritonitis have been reported. Corrosive injury of the eyes may occur. The ingestion of high phosphate products which cause a reduction in ionic calcium may result in tetany.

Treatment: Cationic detergents—Emesis or lavage is contraindicated if a concentrated solution (more than 20%) has been ingested. In these instances, treat as an alkali (see p. 30). Activated charcoal (p. 4) can be used. If a concentration less than 20% has been ingested, induce emesis (Ipecac Syrup, p. 3) or perform gastric lavage (p. 4). Supportive measures for respiratory depresssion, seizures, and vascular collapse may be required. If detergent gets into the eyes, irrigate with water for 15 minutes (p. 6) and consider an examination by an ophthalmologist. Anionic and nonionic detergents are unlikely to be toxic if no spontaneous vomiting occurs within 1 hour. Emesis can be induced (p. 3) if an unusually large amount of detergent has been ingested. If detergent gets into the eyes, irrigate with water for 15 minutes (p. 6). Detergent granules and non-phosphate detergents may require treatment similar to alkali (p. 30).

References:

Feldman, M., Iben, A.B., and Hurley, E.J.: Corrosive injury to oropharynx and esophagus. Eighty-five consecutive cases. California Med., 118:6, January, 1973.

Arena, J.M.: Poisoning and other health hazards associated with use of detergents. J.A.M.A., 190:56, 1964.

Task Group of The Soap and Detergent Association's Biomedical Research Committee: Cleaning Products and Their Accidental Ingestion, ed. 5. New York: The Soap and Detergent Association, 1980.

Grant, W.: Toxicology of the Eye, ed. 2. Springfield, Illinois: Charles C Thomas, pp. 962-967, 1974.

Digitalis and Digitalis Glycosides

Type of Product: Cardiac stimulant.

Ingredients/Description: Digitalis is provided both in tablets and liquid. Digoxin is now the most commonly used cardiac glycoside. Digoxin liquid contains 0.05 mg/ml. Digoxin tablets contain 0.125, 0.25, or 0.5 mg.

Toxicity: Children tolerate relatively larger doses and higher plasma levels of digitalis than adults. The single, lethal, oral dose of all the digitalis glycosides is probably 20 to 50 times the daily maintenance dose. The onset and duration of toxicity varies with the preparation, but half-life varies with the rapidity of loading and the plasma level. Chronic overdose leads to hypokalemia, and acute overdose leads to hyperkalemia. The overlap between toxic and therapeutic doses of the digitalis glycosides is shown in Table 10.

Symptoms: See Table 10.

Treatment: Induce emesis (Ipecac Syrup, p. 3), or perform a gastric lavage (p. 4). Administer orally or by tube a steroid-

Table 10
Symptoms

Grade	Symptoms	Plasma Level (ng/ml)	
		Digoxin	Digitoxin
Nontoxic	None.	0.2-1.5	4-25
Slight	Anorexia, bradycardia, ectopic beats.	1.5-5	25-45
Moderate	Nausea, vomiting, headache, ventricular premature contractions.	5-15	35-55
Severe	Diarrhea, blurring of vision, somnolence, confusion, ventricular tachycardia, sinoatrial or atrioventricular block, hyperkalemia.	10-30	50-80
Extreme	Abdominal pain, convulsions, coma, high-degree conduction blocks, atrial or ventricular fibrillation, severe hyperkalemia.	25-45	>60

Table 11
Treatment of Arrhythmias

Therapy	Indication	Contraindication
Phenytoin (Dilantin), 75 mg/M², IV, every 5 min until ECG response or five doses (typical plasma level 4-20 mg/l) or 600 mg/M²/PO day 1, then 300 mg/M²/PO day 2.	Ventricular premature contractions (including bigeminy, trigeminy, quadrigeminy), ventricular tachycardia; atrial tachycardia with block.	Little value in atrioventricular junctional tachycardia.
Potassium (caution), 0.2-0.6 mEq/min/M², IV, requires 120-160 mEq K/liter in 5% glucose or saline until serum K = 4.0.	Ventricular tachycardia or atrial tachycardia with block only if serum K⁺ <4.0 (dangerous if serum K⁺ normal or elevated).	Atrioventricular block associated with atrial rate <100, unless serum K⁺ <3.0. Sinoatrial or ventricular delay in conduction.

binding resin such as cholestyramine or colestipol to bind any residual digitalis and that which is recirculated enterohepatically. If a resin is not available, give 10 to 20 gm of activated charcoal (0.25 mg digoxin may be adsorbed by 2.0 gm of charcoal). This procedure should be repeated every 6 to 8 hours until the blood level is no longer in the toxic range. Monitor cardiac status with continuous electrocardiograms. Monitor clinical status by immediate and serial assay of plasma digoxin or digitoxin levels and potassium, other electrolytes and blood gases, and indices of renal function. Establish an intravenous line; and, if there is evidence of severe toxicity, consider a central venous monitor.

For treatment of arrhythmias, see Table 11. **Note:** the value of potassium therapy has been overemphasized. Although potassium deficiency increases the binding of ouabain to the myocardium, the overwhelming inhibition of ATPase leads to hyperkalemia. A slight increase in potassium ion speeds atrioventricular conduction, but a greater elevation halves the amount of digitalis needed to produce atrioventricular block. Experience has not made clear a role for hemoperfusion.

Treatment of Hyperkalemia: See Table 12.

If serum potassium is 5.0 to 6.0 mEq/l, administer intravenously 5% or 10% glucose plus sodium bicarbonate as needed.

If serum potassium is 6.0 mEq/l (despite the administration of glucose), administer 0.2 U/kg insulin with 200 to 400 mg/kg glucose; also administer 2 mEq/kg sodium bicarbonate intravenously. Give a Kayexalate retention enema (25% in 25% sorbitol), 1 gm/kg, every 4 to 6 hours.

If serum potassium is 8.0 mEq/l (despite vigorous therapy), hemodialysis or peritoneal dialysis may be indicated (does not remove digitalis).

Investigational: Digoxin-specific FAB antibody fragments in a multi-center study in various population centers around the United States have been used to treat 26 patients with

Table 12
Treatment of Hyperkalemia

Therapy	Indication	Contraindication
Atropine, 0.1 mg/kg, IV or SC, every 4 hr.	Atrioventricular or sinoatrial block, sinus bradycardia, atrial fibrillation with bradycardia.	Ventricular premature contractions or ventricular tachycardia.
Procainamide, 5 mg/kg, IM, every 4-6 hr.	Ventricular premature contractions or ventricular tachycardia unresponsive to potassium.	Sinoatrial or atrioventricular block.
Transvenous pacemaker ventricular.	Bradycardia. Unresponsive to atropine; during drug treatment of ventricular arrhythmia.	Sinoatrial or atrioventricular block.

advanced, life-threatening digoxin (23 cases) or digitoxin (3 cases) toxicity. Success was achieved in 21 patients. Supplies of the FAB fragments at present are limited but offer promise in the future to reverse advanced, life-threatening digitalis intoxication.

References:

Bazzano, G., and Bazzano, G.S.: Digitalis intoxication. Treatment with a new steroid-binding resin. J.A.M.A., **220**:828, 1972.

Bigger, J.T., Jr., and Strauss, H.S.: Digitalis toxicity: Drug interactions promoting toxicity and the management of toxicity. Semin. Drug Treat., **2**:147, Autumn, 1972.

deMicheli, A., Medrano, G.A., Villarreal, A., and Sodi-Pallares, D.: Superiority of the glucose-potassium-insulin solution over the glucose, glucose-insulin and glucose-potassium solutions in acute experimental digitalis intoxication. Acta Cardiol. (Brux), **26**:400, 1971.

Smith, T.W.: Radioimmunoassay for serum Digitoxin concentration: Methodology and clinical experience. J. Pharmacol. Exp. Ther., **175**:352, 1970.

Iacuone, J.J.: Accidental digitoxin poisoning. Amer. J. Dis. Child., **130**:425, 1976.

Schwartz, H.S.: Digitalis intoxication and poisoning. J. Amer. Coll. Emerg. Phys., **6**:168, 1977.

Smith, T.W., Butler, V.P., Haber, E., Fozzard, H., Marcus, F.I., Bremner, F., Schulman, I.C., and Phillips, A.: Treatment of life-threatening digitalis intoxication with digoxin-specific FAB antibody fragments. New Engl. J. Med., **307**:1357, 1982.

Doherty, J.E.: Digoxin antibodies and digitalis intoxication. New Engl. J. Med., **307**:1398, 1982.

Donnatal Products

Type of Product: Antispasmodic.

Manufacturer: A. H. Robins Company.

Ingredients/Description: See Table 13. The belladonna alkaloid content per unit listed in tablets, elixir, capsules, and #2 is equivalent to 0.24 mg of atropine. The atropine equivalent of one Extentab is 0.72 mg. Note: There are a number of other gastrointestinal anticholinergic combination products made by a variety of companies containing belladonna alkaloids, atropine, and barbitals with similar and greater amounts of ingredients.

Toxicity: As little as 10 mg of atropine has been fatal in a child. The estimated fatal dose of atropine is 100 mg, but adult patients have survived this dose in isolated instances. Phenobarbital is potentially fatal for adults at a dose of 5 gm.

Symptoms and Findings: Atropine overdose can cause dilated pupils; dry mouth (thirst, difficulty in swallowing); hyperthermia; flushed, hot, dry skin; headache; nausea; delirium; convulsions; rapid pulse and respiration; and urinary retention. Barbiturates may produce severe central nervous system depression, possibly progressing to coma with respiratory and circulatory failure (see Barbiturates and Atropine, p. 40 and 39).

Treatment: Induce emesis (Ipecac Syrup, p. 3) or perform gastric lavage (p. 4). Decontaminate the lower gastrointestinal tract (p. 5). Prevent hypoxia by use of intubation, respiratory support, and oxygen as needed. Maintain blood pressure with intravenous fluids and vasopressors (dopamine or metaraminol) as needed. Adequate facilities for respiratory support are essential. Forced alkaline diuresis as well as peritoneal or hemodialysis may be indicated in severe phenobarbital overdose (see Barbiturates, p. 40). Symptomatic improvement of atropine effects may be achieved with physostigmine. Physostigmine, which may be

Table 13
Ingredients, Donnatal Products

Ingredient	Tablets, Capsules, Elixir*	Donnatal #2	Extentabs
Hyoscyamine SO$_4$	0.1 mg	0.1 mg	0.3 mg
Atropine SO$_4$	0.02 mg	0.02 mg	0.06 mg
Hyoscine HBr	0.007 mg	0.007 mg	0.02 mg
Phenobarbital	16.20 mg	32.4 mg	48.6 mg

*Elixir only, 23% ethanol.

used for a diagnostic trial, rapidly reverses symptoms of anticholinergic poisoning. Convulsions, hyperthermia, severe tachycardia, coma, and hypertension are all indications for the therapeutic use of physostigmine. Hallucinations may also be an indication if the patient may harm himself or others. Be aware that physostigmine is rapidly destroyed, and the patient's symptoms may return within 1 to 2 hours. The physostigmine dose in children, start with 0.5 mg, slowly intravenously, over 1 minute. Repeat this dose at 5- to 10-minute intervals until reversal of the toxic effects or a maximum of 2 mg is attained. In adults, start with 1 mg, slowly intravenously, over 1 to 3 minutes, and repeat this dose at 5- to 10-minute intervals until reversal of the toxic effects or a maximum of 4 mg is attained. The lowest effective dose should be repeated if life-threatening signs recur.

Neostigmine is ineffective in reversing the effects of atropine on the central nervous system.

References:

Mann, J.B., and Sandberg, D.H.: Therapy of sedative overdosage. Pediat. Clin. N. Amer., **17**:617, 1970.

National Clearinghouse for Poison Control Centers, Washington, D.C., card file index, May 1970.

Rumack, B.H.: Anticholinergic poisoning: Treatment with physostigmine. Pediatrics, **52**:449, 1973.

Also see references for Atropine (p. 40) and Barbiturates (p. 45).

Ethchlorvynol (Placidyl)

Type of Product: Nonbarbiturate hypnotic.

Manufacturer: Abbott Laboratories.

Ingredients/Description: Capsules contain 100, 200, 500, and 750 mg ethchlorvynol (Placidyl).

Toxicity: Patients have survived 60 gm doses, although one adult died after 2.5 gm. Alcohol may augment toxicity. The patient may have extended coma because of an apparently long (100 hour) half-life from an overdose. Withdrawal syndromes (including in the neonate) have been described and require specialized treatment management.

Symptoms and Findings: Central nervous system depression, with profound coma and a flat electroencephalogram may be seen in patients who subsequently recover. Respirations may be depressed. Hypothermia and hypotension with relative bradycardia are common. Peripheral neuropathy has been observed., Pulmonary edema, which is not explained on a cardiodynamic basis, has been seen after both oral and intravenous routes of exposure.

Treatment: Induce emesis (Ipecac Syrup, p. 3), unless the patient is obtunded, or perform gastric lavage (p. 4). Decontaminate the lower gastrointestinal tract (p. 5). Even if the patient has ingested a low dose, a period of observation should follow. Prevent hypoxia by use of intubation and respiratory support as needed. Maintain blood pressure with intravenous fluids and vasopressors (dopamine and metaraminol) as needed. Use cautious warming to restore normal body temperature. Peritoneal dialysis and diuresis are not helpful. Oxygen and positive pressure ventilation may be used if pulmonary edema occurs.

References:

Teehan, B.P., Maher, J.F., Carey, J.H., Flynn, P.D., and Schreiner, G.E.: Acute ethchlorvynol (Placidyl) intoxication. Ann. Intern. Med., **72**:875, 1970.

Glauser, F.L., Smith, W.R., Caldwell, A., Hoshiko, M., Dolan, G.S., Baer, H., and Olsher, N.: Ethchlorvynol (Placidyl)-induced pulmonary edema. Ann. Intern. Med., **84**:46, 1976.

Van Swearingen, P.: Placidyl and pulmonary edema. Ann. Intern. Med., **84**:614, 1976.

Rumack, B.H., and Walravens, P.A.: Neonatal withdrawal following maternal ingestion of ethchlorvynol (Placidyl). Pediatrics, **52**:714, 1973.

Ethyl Alcohol

Type of Product: Beverages; solvents for perfumes and colognes; ingredient of some aftershave lotions, mouthwashes, liniments, tinctures; ingredient of some rubbing alcohols.

Ingredients: Whiskey, 40 to 50% alcohol (80 to 100 proof); liqueurs, 22 to 50% alcohol; wines, 10 to 14% alcohol; beer,

3 to 8% alcohol. Colognes may be 40 to 60% alcohol. Alcohol in cosmetics (including colognes) is denatured, but the denaturant does not contribute significantly to the toxicity unless it is methyl alcohol.

Toxicity: The following symptoms are caused by depression of the brain by ethanol and are related to serum concentration:

50-100 mg/dl (mg%)	socially "high"
100-200 mg/dl (mg%)	intoxicated
200-400 mg/dl (mg%)	moderate to severe intoxication
400-500 mg/dl (mg%)	about the LD_{50} for nonalcohol-dependent adults
800 mg/dl (mg%) and up	few survive

Serum levels can be estimated from dose, particularly when the ethanol is ingested over a short time. Calculations are made in terms of 100% alcohol. One milliliter per kilogram will give a serum level of more than 100 mg% (mg/dl). In those who have been drinking over a period of time, food and the time course of ingestion make the foregoing estimation less reliable. The rate of metabolism for ethyl alcohol is approximately 125 mg/kg per hour (see p. 15).

In the laboratory, blood ethanol concentrations are best done by gas-liquid chromatography to differentiate the presence of other alcohols. When absolutely certain that ethanol alone has been ingested, an enzymatic assay for blood ethanol concentrations is adequate. Serum osmolality determined by freezing-point depression may also be useful; a rise in plasma osmolality of 21.7 mOm/kg H_2O reflects an increase of 100 mg/100 ml in plasma alcohol. Determined osmolality will exceed calculated serum osmolality (see p. 14 for formula for calculations). Ethanol is metabolized as follows:

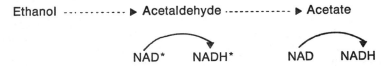

Ethanol ----------▶ Acetaldehyde ------------▶ Acetate

NAD*   NADH*   NAD   NADH

---

*NAD = nicotinamide-adenine dinucleotide; NADH = reduced nicotinamide-adenine dinucleotide.

Two molecules of NAD are used up and rendered unavailable for gluconeogenesis; this may result in hypoglycemia and lacticacidemia, especially with blood levels more than 100 mg% (mg/dl). Hypoglycemia is inceasingly common the younger the child.

Ethyl alcohol is a gastrointestinal tract irritant and may cause repeated vomiting and hematemesis.

Symptoms and Findings: Exhilaration, incoordination, slurred speech, ataxia, nausea, and vomiting with risk of aspiration may occur. Repeated vomiting may add to dehydration and acidemia. A flushed face, sweating, hypothermia, tachycardia, variable pupillary reactions, hypotension, coma, and shock may be present. Hypoglycemia and convulsions occur in all ages. Children are less apt to show exhilaration and are particularly prone to hypoglycemia and convulsions. Withdrawal-type symptoms (including in the neonate) have been described and require specialized treatment management.

Treatment: Induce emesis (Ipecac Syrup, p. 3) or perform gastric lavage (p. 4) with sodium bicarbonate (3 to 5% solution). In children, serum glucose determinations should be made. If a known amount of 1 ml/kg 100% alcohol or more or an unknown amount was ingested, the concentration of alcohol in the serum must be determined. Protect against aspiration. Prevent hypoxia by use of intubation, respiratory support, and oxygen as needed. Correct hypothermia and maintain body temperature. Maintain on intravenous fluids to correct hypoglycemia and lacticacidemia. Hypotension should be treated with plasma expanders, fluids, and pressors. In young children, if the serum concentration is 300 mg% (mg/dl) or more, consider peritoneal dialysis or hemodialysis.

References:

Sellers, E.M., and Kalant, H.: Alcohol intoxication and withdrawal. New Engl. J. Med., 294:757, 1976.

Leake, C.D., and Silverman, M.: Chemistry of alcoholic beverages. *In* Kissin, B., and Begleiter, H., ed.: The Biology of Alcoholism, Vol. 1. New York: Plenum Press, pp. 575-610, 1971.

Cummins, J.H.: Hypoglycemia and convulsions in children following alcohol ingestion. J. Pediat., 58:23, 1961.

Pierog, S., Chandavasu, O., and Wexler, I.: Withdrawal symptoms in infants with fetal alcohol syndrome. J. Pediat., 90:630, 1977.

Cook, L.N., Shott, R.J., and Andrews, B.F.: Acute transplacental ethanol intoxication. Amer. J. Dis. Child., **129**:1075, 1975.

Vasiliades, J.: Emergency toxicology: The evaluation of three analytical methods for the determination of misused alcohols. Clin. Toxicol., **10**:399, 1977.

Beard, J.D., Knott, D.H., and Fink, R.D.: The use of plasma and urine osmolality in evaluating the acute phase of alcohol abuse. South. Med. J., **67**:271, 1974.

Ethylene Glycol

Type of Product: Main ingredient in permanent-type antifreeze.

Ingredients/Description: Colorless liquid with a faint odor and an acrid-sweet taste.

Toxicity: Death in adults has been reported from the ingestion of 100 ml (1.4 ml/kg). Inhalation and skin absorption are possible but unlikely routes of toxicity. Manifestations of toxicity are mainly related to the metabolites of ethylene glycol, although the parent compound may cause initial cerebral depresssion, and a small amount may be excreted in the urine unchanged. Metabolism proceeds via NAD-dependent enzymes to aldehydes and glycolic, glyoxylic and formic acids, which may lead to a fairly rapid onset of acidosis. The ultimate pathway is the formation of oxalic acid and the resulting oxalate crystals precipitated in the kidney, which may cause renal failure. The oxalate formation may be intensified by the depletion of pyridoxine in the presence of excessive amounts of glyoxylate as the metabolic breakdown of ethylene glycol proceeds. Renal damage may also be caused by the other metabolites.

Symptoms and Findings: Clinical finding may progress in three stages. The first stage, which has its onset within 30 minutes to 12 hours, is primarily one of intoxication, with ataxia, nausea, vomiting, and abdominal pain; and, depending on dose, it may progress to stupor, coma, and convulsions. Low grade fever and tachycardia may be observed. Papilledema, nystagmus, or ophthalmoplegia have been reported rarely. Pleocytosis has been found in the spinal fluid, and leukocytosis has been observed in the blood. Laboratory findings may reveal severe metabolic acidosis, a large anion gap, and increased measured osmolality over calculated osmolality. The second stage may be fairly indistinct, and cardiopulmonary symptoms may become prominent. These may be congestive heart failure or pulmonary edema. Hypocalcemia exacerbates the toxicity on the heart. Skeletal muscle pain with elevated blood creatinine phosphokinase levels have been reported. The third stage is primarily one of renal involvement. The earliest indication may be manifest by CVA tenderness, the finding of calcium oxalate and hippurate crystals in the urine, or the development of varying degrees of renal impairment. Acute tubular necrosis has been reported as early as 12 hours postingestion. Recovery has occurred after prolonged oliguria. Rarely, optic atrophy has been observed.

Treatment: Induce emesis (Ipecac Syrup, p. 3) or perform gastric lavage (p. 4). Prevent hypoxia by use of intubation, respiratory support, and oxygen as needed. Obtain electrolyte, arterial blood gas, and BUN determinations. Obtain ethylene glycol levels if available. Correct acidosis with intravenous fluids and sodium bicarbonate (3 to 5 mEq/kg). Correct hypocalcemia (below 8.5 mEq/100 ml) with 10 ml of a 10% calcium gluconate solution, administered slowly intravenously. Monitor urine output, specific gravity, proteinuria, and miscroscopic crystals and cells. Attempt to maintain adequate urine output with intravenous fluids and furosemide or mannitol (contraindicated if oliguria with crystalluria is present). If the patient is in the first stage of the intoxication, initiate ethanol therapy (p. 15); the route depends on the patient's clinical status. The goal is to create a blood ethanol level of 100 to 150 mg% (mg/dl) to saturate alcohol dehydrogenase in the liver and prevent further metabolism of the ethylene glycol (p. 15). As with methanol, ethylene glycol will be eliminated in the urine when hepatic metabolism is blocked by ethanol. The loading dose of ethanol is approximately 1 ml of 100% alcohol (0.79 gm) per kilogram; the maintenance dose is based on the calculated rate of metabolism of ethanol (approximately 125 mg/kg per hour). If it is given intravenously, ethanol should be diluted to 5 to 10%, usually in D_5W. Ethanol blood levels must be monitored, and ethanol administration must be continued for at least 24 hours, or until ethylene glycol is removed from the body. In a severe overdose, with blood ethylene glycol levels of 50 mg/dl or more, severe metabolic acidosis, or renal failure, institute hemodialysis (preferably) or peritoneal dialysis while continuing on ethanol therapy.[1] Protect against hypoglycemia with glucose administration. Replacement of pyridoxine may be salutory. Treat shock, coma, and convulsions.

References:

Parry, M.F., and Wallach, R.: Ethylene glycol poisoning. Amer. J. Med.,**57**:143, 1974.

Clay, K.L., and Murphy, R.C.: On the metabolic acidosis of ethylene glycol intoxication. Toxicol. Appl. Pharmacol., **39**:39, 1977.

Tintinalli, J.E.: Of anions, osmols, and methanol poisoning. J. Amer. Coll. Emerg. Phys., **6**:417, 1977.

Peterson, C.D., Collins, A.J., Himes, J.M., Bullock, M.D., and Keane, W.F.: Ethylene glycol poisoning. Pharmacokinetics during therapy with ethanol and hemodialysis. New Engl. J. Med., **304**:21, 1981.

Glutethimide (Doriden)

Type of Product: Nonbarbiturate sedative.

Manufacturer: USV Pharmaceutical Corporation makes Doriden. Several companies manufacture glutethimide.

Ingredients/Description: Doriden tablets contain 125, 250, and 500 mg, and the capsules contain 500 mg of glutethimide.

Toxicity: Ingestion of 5 gm by adults leads to serious complications, and ingestions of more than 10 gm or 0.15 gm/kg have been associated with a significant mortality rate. The drug is fat stored, and its metabolite is also active in prolonging the duration of the effects. The effects are exaggerated by the presence of hypnotics or sedatives.

Symptoms and Findings: Symptoms include central nervous system depression, frequently with fluctuations in consciousness, but progressing to profound coma with fixed, dilated pupils and papilledema; hypotension that may be

---

1. McCoy, H.G., Cipolle, R.J. Ehlers, S.M., Sawchuk, R.J., and Zaske, D.E.: Severe methanol poisoning. Application of a pharmacokinetic model for ethanol therapy and hemodialysis. Amer. J. Med., **67**:804, 1979.

unresponsive to volume expansion but is possibly improved by large doses of steroids; sudden apnea without gradual respiratory depression; hypothermia sometimes followed by hyperpyrexia, muscle twitchings; convulsions. In children, fever, dry mucous membranes, flushing, and ataxia may mimic atropine poisoning.

Treatment: Induce emesis (Ipecac Syrup, p. 3) or perform gastric lavage (p. 4), followed by decontamination of the lower gastrointestinal tract (p. 5). Maintain body temperature. Prevent hypoxia by use of intubation, respiratory support, and oxygen as needed. Maintain blood pressure with intravenous fluids and vasopressors (dopamine or metaraminol) as needed. Forced diuresis is of no value. Dialysis may be used to correct electrolyte imbalance. Most patients will recover with good supportive care.

References:

Hansen, A.R., Kennedy, K.A., Ambre, J.J., and Fischer, L.J.: Glutethimide poisoning. A metabolite contributes to morbidity and mortality. New Engl. J. Med., **292**:250, 1975.

Wright, N., and Roscoe, P.: Acute glutethimide poisoning. Conservative management of 31 patients. J.A.M.A., **214**:1704, 1970.

Myers, R.R., and Stockard, J.J.: Neurologic and electroencephalographic correlates in glutethimide intoxication. Clin. Pharm. Toxicol., **17**:212, 1975.

Hydrogen Peroxide

Type of Product: Oxidizing agent.

Ingredients/Description: Hydrogen peroxide is an oxidizing liquid marketed as aqueous solutions of different common concentrations: 3% in a topical antiseptic, 6% in hair preparations (bleaches, neutralizers, and so forth), 30% for industrial and laboratory use, and 90% for use in rocket propulsion.

Toxicity: The industrial strengths may be corrosive. No primary systemic effects are noted when less than 10% solutions are ingested because it decomposes to oxygen in the bowel before absorption.

Symptoms and Findings: Decomposition of hydrogen peroxide may release large volumes of oxygen (10 times the volume for a 3% solution). Rupture of the colon, proctitis, and ulcerative colitis have been reported after hydrogen peroxide enemas. Suffocation from foam may occur with highly concentrated solutions. Dropping a 3% solution on the eye three to five times a day has been reported to be innocuous. A high concentration of hydrogen peroxide has the potential to cause severe corneal damage. Ingestion of the commonly available household products (3 to 6%) should cause no problem other than possible mucous membrane and gastrointestinal irritation. Higher concentrations may cause corrosive lesions of the mucous membranes, the eye, and the skin.

Treatment: Dilute the ingested product with a glass of milk or water. Flush the eyes thoroughly with water (p. 6). If a high concentration was ingested, treat as under alkali (p. 30). Provide symptomatic and supportive treatment otherwise.

References:

Gosselin, R.E., Hodge, H.C., Smith, R.P., and Gleason, M.N.: Clinical Toxicology of Commercial Products: Acute Poisoning, ed. 4. Baltimore: Williams and Wilkins, Section II, p. 74, 1976, reprinted 1977.

Grant, W.M.: Toxicology of the Eye, ed. 2. Springfield, Illinois: Charles C Thomas, pp. 559-560, 1974.

Giusti, G.V.: Fatal poisoning with hydrogen peroxide. Forensic Sci., 2:99, 1973.

Iron Salts

Type of Product: Medicinal preparation for anemia.

Ingredients/Description: See Tables 14 and 15.

Toxicity: The reported, average lethal dose is 180 mg elemental iron per kilogram (0.9 gm ferrous sulfate per kilogram). However, the minimum lethal dose is as little as 600 mg elemental iron (3 gm ferrous sulfate). Total doses of 200 to 400 mg elemental iron have caused severe symptoms in young children. The dosage of elemental iron that is poten-

Table 14
Iron Content of Some Preparations

Salt	Iron Content	Average Tablet Strength	Iron Content per Tablet
Ferrous Sulfate	20%	300 mg	60 mg
Ferrous Sulfate, dried	29.7%	200 mg	65 mg
Ferrous Gluconate	11.6%	320 mg	36 mg
Ferrous Fumarate	33%	200 mg	67 mg
Ferrocholinate	12%	333 mg	40 mg

tially dangerous is unclear but seems to range from 20 to 60 mg/kg. The rate-limiting factor in the gastrointestinal tract for absorption of iron does not seem to work in the presence of a large excess. There is no physiologic mechanism for the excretion of iron except through blood loss or gastrointestinal desquamations. Ferrous and ferric salts may also cause corrosive damage to the stomach and small intestines.

Some iron preparations are radiopaque and can be visualized on an x-ray of the abdomen.

Symptoms and Findings: Acute iron poisoning in children characteristically follows a biphasic course. Usually a portion of the tablets (or liquid) ingested is vomited within one-half hour. Vomitus may be bloody and contain partially digested tablets; vomiting can recur for up to several hours. However, enteric-coated tablets may pass into the small intestine without causing gastric symptoms. (Retained tablets may be visible by x-ray.) Abdominal cramps may or may not occur during the first 6 to 12 hours, then tarry stools or bloody diarrhea, lethargy, and, in severe cases, acidosis and shock may occur. Leukocytosis and fever may also be present. The child may appear to improve clinically after this first symptomatic phase, only to lapse unexpectedly into profound cardiovascular collapse some hours later. This second phase is usually associated with hepatic injury. Latent periods between these two symptomatic phases may last from a few to 48 hours. The course is difficult to predict, but the second stage is not seen in milder cases. Serum iron levels and, if available, total iron-binding capacity within 4 to 6 hours of ingestions are important. Late complications (several weeks to months after the acute episode) of hepatic cirrhosis or pyloric or duodenal stenosis have been reported.

Treatment: The patient may be given milk and observed at home if it can definitely be ascertained that less than one-half the minimal toxic dose of elemental iron has been ingested; the patient has no symptoms; and it is clearly understood that, if vomiting, abdominal pain, diarrhea, black or bloody stools develop, the patient must be seen in the emergency room immediately.

In all patients where one-half or more of the toxic dose of iron-containing compounds have been suspected of having been ingested, emesis should be induced (Ipecac Syrup, p. 3).

When the ingestion of iron is in doubt and may have occurred within the preceding 4 hours, the qualitative deferoxamine color test for iron in gastric contents may be helpful.

If the patient is having hematemesis, is lethargic, or is in shock, gastric lavage should be performed (p. 4). Approximately 100 ml of a 5% sodium bicarbonate solution in water

Table 15
Examples of Multivitamins with Iron

Tablet	Elemental Iron per Tablet
Chocks Plus Iron	15 mg
Chocks Bugs Bunny Plus Iron	15 mg
Flintstones Plus Iron	15 mg
One-a-day Plus Minerals	18 mg
One-a-day Plus Iron	18 mg
Monsters with Iron	12 mg
Pals with Iron	12 mg
Poly-visol with Iron	12 mg
Chronosule	78 mg

should be left in the stomach to convert any free ferrous salt to insoluble ferrous carbonate and hopefully inhibit the local irritative consequences. Although a disodium phosphate solution (Fleet's enema diluted four to one) has also been used instead of sodium bicarbonate, complications have been reported from the use of excessive amounts of a hypertonic phosphate solution. There is no scientific data to support the effectiveness of phosphate over bicarbonate, so the risk from its use should be avoided.

The use of deferoxamine (Desferal mesylate) in the gastro-intestinal tract is controversial. The iron-ferroxamine complex (ferrioxamine) is absorbed and, in dog studies, appears to be toxic. It seems prudent not to use defer-oxamine in this manner until further studies have proven its safety.

The lower gastrointestinal tract also needs to be emptied. If no bleeding is evident, a saline laxative followed by an enema may remove unabsorbed iron tablets. An x-ray of the abdomen may reveal their presence; and, if vomiting and lavage are unsuccessful in removing the tablets, they may need to be surgically removed from the stomach or by enemas from the bowel. When more than a few chewable multivitamins and iron preparations have been taken, abdominal cramps and excessive stools commonly occur spontaneously, and the remaining tablets are probably fully expelled. Chewable multivitamin and iron tablets are not expected to show on an x-ray.

A serum iron level and, if available, a total iron-binding capacity or an iron screen (such as the Fischer test which measures the amount of free iron) should be obtained. There is no clear evidence of the optimal time to obtain the serum iron and the total iron-binding capacity; but it seems reasonable, depending on the form the ingested iron was in and the age of the child, to obtain these levels between 2 to 4 hours after ingestion. A liquid preparation is apt to be absorbed fastest, then chewable multivitamins with iron next, and enteric-coated tablets are the slowest.

Children may have gastrointestinal symptoms for a short period associated with free iron levels under 300 μg%. Black stools should be tested for blood. Few patients develop serious symptoms with a free iron level between 300 and 600 μg%. The levels must be related to the time of ingestion, history, and the patient's clinical presentation. Generally, if the time frame is within the first few hours after ingestion, the history dependable, and the **gastrointestinal tract cleaned out**, a trial of the specific chelator deferoxamine may be given with free iron levels between 300 and 600 μg%. Some advise that a 40 mg/kg intramuscular dose be given; others prefer to administer the drug (0.5 to 1 gm) in an intravenous drip over 4 hours (never to exceed 15 mg/kg per hour to prevent the occurrence of hypotension) and observe for the excretion of the iron-ferroxamine complex, which colors the urine an orange-rose (vin rosé). If the color does not appear by 2 hours after the drip is finished and the patient is asymptomatic, the patient may be discharged (however, one worrisome case of iron poisoning has been reported where the urine never changed color). Patients with levels of 600 μg% or more of free iron, whether asymptomatic or not, should be admitted and treated with deferoxamine. The dose of deferoxamine may need to be repeated every 4 to 6 hours until the color is no longer evident in the urine. Not more than 6 gm of deferoxamine should be given in 24 hours; 100 mg can bind only 8.5 mg of iron, or 6 gm can bind 500 mg.

While the foregoing procedures are taking place, supportive therapy also should be instituted. A type and crossmatch should be drawn at the time of the initial iron level. If metabolic acidosis is present, it should be treated with sodium bicarbonate in an intravenous line separate from the deferoxamine. Shock may require intensive therapy. Demulcents should be administered to protect the upper gastrointestinal tract.

When free serum iron approaches 1,000 μg%, serious consideration must be given to more heroic measures of treatment, hopefully before the patient goes into shock, has a bleeding diathesis, or shows signs of liver toxicity. Peritoneal and hemodialysis have been of little benefit. Exchange transfusion has been used with some success.

Starting deferoxamine after 12 to 18 hours may be of little value. When deferoxamine is indicated, it should be started as soon as possible. The opportunity for a successful outcome diminishes considerably after severe liver damage occurs.

All treated patients should be seen within 2 weeks of discharge to ensure that there are no gastrointestinal symptoms. X-ray examinations of the gastrointestinal tract may be indicated if a stricture is suspected. Anticipate eventual resolution of malabsorption syndromes. Check for iron deficiency from blood loss and/or excessive therapy of the acute illness.

References:

Whitten, C.F., Chen, Y.C., and Gibson, G.W.: Studies in acute iron poisonings. II. Further observations on desferrioxamine in the treatment of acute experimental iron poisoning. Pediatrics, 38:102, 1966.

Fischer, D.S.: A method for the rapid detection of acute iron toxicity. Clin. Chem., 13:6, 1967.

Angle, C.R.: Symposium on iron poisoning. Clin. Toxicol., 4:525, 1971.

Robertson, W.O.: Iron poisoning: A problem of childhood. Topics Emerg. Med., 1:57, No. 3, 1979.

Robotham, J.L., and Lietman, P.S.: Acute iron poisoning: A review. Amer. J. Dis. Child., 134:875, 1980.

Banner, W., Jr., and Czajka, P.A.: Iron poisoning. Amer. J. Dis. Child., 135:484, 1981.

Czajka, P.A., Konrad, J.D., and Duffy, J.P.: Iron poisoning: An in vitro comparison of bicarbonate and phosphate lavage solutions. J. Pediat., 98:491, 1981.

McGuigan, M.A., Lovejoy, F.H., Jr., Marino, S.K., Propper, R.D., and Goldman, P.: Qualitative deferoxamine color test for iron ingestion. J. Pediat., 94:940, 1979.

Isoniazid

Type of Product: Antituberculosis drug.

Manufacturer: INH–CIBA, 300 mg tablets and 150 mg capsules in combination with 300 mg rifampin. Nydrazid–Squibb, 100 mg tablets. Generic–Lilly, McKesson, Purepac, and others.

Ingredients/Description: Tablets of 50, 100, and 300 mg. Injectable form in vials of 10 ml containing 100 mg/ml.

Toxicity: Symptoms occur in adults with the ingestion of 1.5 gm of isoniazed. Doses between 6 and 10 gm are associated with severe symptoms. Death occurred in a 13-year-old child from the ingestion of 3 gm. Symptoms in the central nervous system are produced in part by interruption of neurotransmitter production. Acidosis may be produced by other metabolic blocks and seizure activity.

Symptoms and Findings: The onset of symptoms occurs between 30 and 90 minutes after ingestion. Symptoms and signs progress rapidly and may include nausea, vomiting, blurred vision, visual hallucinations, dizziness, slurred speech, dilated pupils, tachycardia, and urinary retention. These are followed by hyperreflexia, stupor, coma, and generalized or focal seizures. There may also be hyporeflexia, hypotension, and cyanosis. Severe metabolic acidosis, hyperpyrexia, hyperglycemia, hyperkalemia, and albuminuria may occur. Death results from respiratory arrest or circulatory failure.

Treatment: Induce emesis (Ipecac Syrup, p. 3) or perform gastric lavage (p. 4). Be aware of the rapid onset of symptoms. Decontaminate the lower gastrointestinal tract (p. 5). If the patient is asymptomatic, observe for at least 4 hours. Obtain isoniazid level, glucose, electrolytes, bicarbonate, and arterial blood gases. If the patient is symptomatic, prevent hypoxia by use of intubation, respiratory support, and oxygen as needed; start intravenous fluids. Administer pyridoxine HCl (1 gm for each estimated gram of isoniazid ingested) intravenously over 5 minutes. The same dose of pyridoxine HCl may be repeated in comatose or convulsing patients at 5- to 20-minute intervals. If the total dose taken is unknown, initially administer at least 5 gm pyridoxine HCl slowly intravenously. Then, correct acidosis with fluids and sodium bicarbonate (3 to 5 mEq/kg) intravenously as needed. Some clinicians have found that spontaneous correction of acidosis occurs after administration of pyridoxine and cessation of the seizures. If needed, diazepam (0.05 to 0.1 mg/kg, intravenously) may be given initially for seizures. If hypotension occurs, use fluid replacement monitored by central venous pressure measurement. Dialysis is helpful in removing isoniazid, but it is rarely required.

References:

Brown, C.V.: Acute isoniazid poisoning. Amer. Rev. Resp. Dis., **105**:206, 1972.

Miller, J., Robinson, A., and Percy, A.K.: Acute isoniazid poisoning in childhood. Amer. J. Dis. Child., **134**:290, 1980.

Kingston, R.L., and Saxena, K.: Management of acute isoniazid overdosages. Clin. Toxicol. Consultant, **2**:37, 1980.

Cameron, W.M.: Isoniazid overdose. Canad. Med. Assn. J., 118:1413, 1978.

Königshausen, T., Altragge, G., Hein, D., Grabensee, B., and Pütter, D.: Hemodialysis and hemaperfusion in the treatment of most severe INH-poisoning. Veterin. Human Toxicol. (Suppl.), 21:12, 1979.

Wason, S., Lacouture, P.G., and Lovejoy, F.H., Jr.: Single high-dose pyridoxine treatment for isoniazid overdose. J.A.M.A., 246:1102, 1981.

Isopropyl Alcohol

Type of Product: Rubbing alcohol (Check individual product for ingredient percentage).

Ingredients/Description: A clear, colorless liquid found principally in rubbing solutions in various concentrations. It is usually sold in pint bottles, and color may have been added. It is also used as a solvent in some skin lotions and medications and as deicing and antifreeze preparations.

Toxicity: The toxic dose is approximately 1 ml/kg of 70% isopropanol, which will produce a serum level of 70 mg/dl. The central nervous system depressant effects are about twice those of ethyl alcohol at comparable blood levels. Serum levels more than 50 mg/dl are an indication for close observation of the patient. Peak serum levels usually are reached in 1 hour and may not fall as rapidly as ethyl alcohol levels because isopropyl alcohol is secreted back from blood through the salivary glands and the stomach. Hypoglycemia may occur because of the use of NAD in alcohol metabolism and the resultant diminution of gluconeogenesis (see Ethanol, p. 68). Some isopropyl alcohol is excreted unchanged by the lungs and the kidneys, but most of it is metabolized by alcohol dehydrogenase in the liver to acetone, which spills in the urine and may be smelled on the breath.

Toxicity may occur from inhalation of high concentrations, and deep coma has been reported from sponging a febrile child. Isopropyl alcohol is also absorbed rectally.

Symptoms and Findings: There may be an acute onset of central nervous system depression, manifest as dizziness, headache, incoordination, stupor, or coma. It is more irritating to the gastrointestinal tract than ethyl alcohol, and it is likely to produce vomiting, hematemesis, and diarrhea. The patient may develop hypothermia, bradycardia, hypotension, and even circulatory collapse. Symptoms may persist two to four times longer than with ethyl alcohol ingestion. Acetonuria, ketosis, and anuria may occur. Pulmonary damage and edema may occur as a result of pulmonary excretion of the alcohol. Hypoglycemia occurs, particularly in small children. An increased osmolal gap associated with a high serum acetone, a normal blood pH, a normal serum bicarbonate level, and a normal anion gap is characteristic of isopropyl alcohol intoxication.

Treatment: Usually treatment is required only if more than 5 ml is ingested. Induce emesis (Ipecac Syrup, p. 3) or perform gastric lavage (p. 4). Administer activated charcoal (p. 4). Maintain pulmonary ventilation and blood pressure. Treat hypothermia. Obtain blood for an isopropanol concentration, acetone level, glucose level, and arterial pH. If the patient is hypoglycemic, administer 50% glucose intravenously. Forced water diuresis is not effective; however, osmotic diuresis with hypertonic glucose may increase renal clearance of isopropyl alcohol. If the isopropyl alcohol serum level is 150 mg/dl (mg%) or above, or the patient has hypotension unresponsive to intravenous fluids, peritoneal dialysis or hemodialysis may be life saving.

If an analysis of the isopropanol serum concentration is not available, a useful estimate of the serum concentration can be made by calculating from the increase of serum osmolarity above that predicated from serum electrolytes. Send serum for electrolytes, BUN, glucose, and osmolarity **determined by freezing-point depression.**

$$\text{Calculated mOsm} = \frac{1.86 \times (\text{Na}) + \frac{(\text{glucose})}{18} + \frac{(\text{Serum Urea N})}{2.8}}{0.93}$$

$$\text{Measured mOsm} - \text{Calculated mOsm} = \Delta\text{mOsm}$$

$$\frac{\Delta\text{mOsm} \times 58 \text{ (mol weight of isopropanol)}}{10} = \text{mg/dl of isopropanol.}$$

The serum acetone level usually rises as the serum isopropanol level drops. Gastric drainage or repeated gastric lavage, as long as the patient is comatose, may remove additional isopropyl alcohol. Treatment for gastritis should be instituted. Kidney and liver function tests may be abnormal and should be evaluated for possible long-term sequelae.

References:

McFadden, S.W., and Haddow, J.E.: Coma produced by topical application of isopropanol. Pediatrics, 43:622, 1969.

Dua, S.L.: Peritoneal dialysis for isopropyl alcohol poisoning. J.A.M.A., 230:35, 1974.

King, L.H., Jr., Bradley, K.P., and Shires, D.L., Jr.: Hemodialysis for isopropyl alcohol poisoning. J.A.M.A., 211:1855, 1970.

Agarwal, S.K.: Non-acidotic acetonemia: A syndrome due to isopropyl alcohol intoxication. J. Med. Soc. N.J., 76:914, 1979.

Vasiliades, J.: Emergency toxicology: The evaluation of three analytical methods for the determination of misused alcohols. Clin. Toxicol., 10:399, 1977.

Kerosene and Related Petroleum Distillates

Type of Product: Solvents, fuels, cleaning agents, polishes, diluents, lighter fluids.

Ingredients/Description (in order of decreasing volatility): Petroleum ether (Benzine), petroleum naphtha, mineral seal oil contained in furniture polish, gasoline, petroleum mineral spirits, kerosene, and lubricating oil.

Toxicity: Most deaths following ingestion of kerosene and petroleum distillates are the result of pulmonary effects. Products with low viscosity (30 to 60 SSU), such as lighter fuels, have a high aspiration hazard because of their tendency to spread over a large surface area such as the lungs. Chemical pneumonia results from aspiration of as little as a few milliliters, which usually occurs at the time of ingestion or eructation, particularly in young children. Much larger amounts can be tolerated by ingestion if the product is not aspirated. Systemic absorption of these substances may produce central nervous system, cardiac, renal, hematological, and gastrointestinal effects. Petroleum distillates with high viscosity (150 to 250 SSU) — such as tar, motor oil, transmission oil, cutting oil, household oil, fuel oil, diesel oil, mineral oil, petrolatum, and heavy greases —

have a limited toxicity manifested by minimal gastroenteritis or, if aspirated, by lipoid pneumonia.

Symptoms and Findings: Ingestions may produce a burning sensation of the mouth and esophagus; there may be vomiting and diarrhea. Either inhalation or ingestion may cause euphoria, a burning sensation of the chest and mucous membranes, headache, tinnitus, vertigo, nausea, restlessness, weakness, visual disturbance, incoordination, confusion, central nervous system depression with or without convulsions, peripheral cyanosis, and death from respiratory arrest. Chemical pneumonia is indicated by cough, fever, rapid breathing, cyanosis, tachycardia, and pulmonary edema. A chest x-ray is the best diagnostic tool for pneumonitis, but it may not show changes for 6 to 8 hours after the aspiration. Secondary bacterial infection, albuminuria, hemolysis, hepatosplenomegaly, and cardiac dilatation, flutter, or failure infrequently occur. Many petroleum distillates are gastric irritants. Gasoline can cause second degree skin burns if it is not promptly washed off.

Treatment: Usually, only small amounts of petroleum distillates are inadvertently or accidentally ingested and/or aspirated. Therefore, emesis and gastric lavage should not be used in most instances. Emesis (Ipecac Syrup, p. 3) is indicated only in an alert patient without respiratory distress who is known to have ingested: (1) a petroleum distillate with a concomitant toxic chemical such as heavy metals, pesticides, nitrobenzene, and aniline (check for methemoglobinemia with the latter two chemicals). (2) more than 1 ml/kg of kerosene or gasoline. Do not induce emesis in a patient with respiratory distress, with central nervous system depresssion, or in a coma, or when vomiting has already occurred.

Gastric lavage (p. 4) should be used for unusual circumstances, such as comatose patients, particularly when a more toxic poison is dissolved in the petroleum distillate. Prior to gastric lavage, it is advisable to have a snug-fitting endotracheal tube inserted if it can be done by someone expert in the technique.

A chest x-ray may be positive within 15 minutes of ingestion, but it usually does not correlate with the clinical picture for several hours. Patients with respiratory distress should be admitted without delay. The asymptomatic patient should be observed for 6 to 8 hours. Hospitalization may be indicated if clinical symptoms develop over the observation period or if pulmonary x-ray findings worsen.

Antibiotics do not change the course of chemical pneumonitis, but they are indicated for secondary bacterial infections. Diagnosis of secondary bacterial pneumonia is assisted by an increased white blood cell count and a recurrence of fever.

Corticosteroids are of no proven value. Epinephrine and norepinephrine are contraindicated because they may precipitate cardiac arrhythmias.

Pneumatoceles may be found on follow-up chest x-rays after the patient has clinically recovered. The pneumatoceles usually spontaneously disappear in days to weeks without any intervention.

References:

Gerarde, H.W.: Toxicological studies on hydrocarbons. IX. The aspiration hazard and toxicity of hydrocarbons and hydrocarbon mixtures. Arch. Environ. Health, 6:329, 1963.

Ng, R.C., Darwish, H., and Stewart, D.A.: Emergency treatment of petroleum distillate and turpentine ingestion. Canad. Med. Assn. J., 111:537, 1974.

Bratton, L., and Haddow, J.E.: Ingestion of charcoal lighter fluid. J. Pediat., 87:633, 1975.

Mann, M.D., Pirie, D.J., and Wolfsdorf, J.: Kerosene absorption in primates. J. Pediat., 91:495, 1977.

Brown, J., III, Burke, B., and Dajani, A.S.: Experimental kerosene pneumonia: Evaluation of some therapeutic regimens. J. Pediat., 84:396, 1974.

Bergeson, P.S., Hales, S.W., Lustgarten, M.D., and Lipow, H.W.: Pneumatoceles following hydrocarbon ingestion. Report of three cases and review of the literature. Amer. J. Dis. Child., 129:49, 1975.

Anas, N., Namasonthi, V., and Ginsburg, C.M.: Criteria for hospitalizing children who have ingested products containing hydrocarbons. J.A.M.A., 246:840, 1981.

Rumack, B.H.: Hydrocarbon ingestions in perspective. J. Amer. Coll. Emerg. Phys., 6:172, 1977.

Lead

Type of Product: Paint; objects made of lead; tetraethyl lead gasoline additive; dust from smelters; fumes from molten lead, burning old paint, or lead plates; unvented kilns.

Sources: Lead poisoning results most commonly from repetitive absorption of lead from the gastrointestinal tract. Acute poisoning is exceptionally rare. There are a few case reports from a single, massive, oral dose of lead salts or from the inhalation of lead vapors. The chronic course of poisoning may be punctuated by acute symptomatic episodes. If metallic lead objects (e.g., fishing sinkers, toy soldiers, costume jewelry) are retained in the stomach, they will dissolve and release lead slowly so acute symptoms of poisoning may begin after 1 to 2 months. The glaze and frit on some ceramic dishes and containers that have been inadequately fired may release lead in the presence of acidic foods. Illicit whiskey can contain enough lead to cause lead posioning. Automotive exhausts contain lead in an inorganic form. The concentrations of lead in air, except in unusual circumstances, are insufficient to produce clinical poisoning. Lead dusts may be brought home on shoes and clothing by the unthinking worker and contaminate house dust. Organic lead (lead naphthenate or tetraethyl lead) exposure is generally limited to industrial exposure or intentional inhalation abuse.

Overexposure to lead varies with age. In the young child, increased lead absorption results most commonly from repetitive ingestion of old paint, old putty, and lead-contaminated dirt and dust.

In older children and adolescents in whom pica — except in retarded children — can be excluded, alternate sources should be checked (i.e., lead objects retained in the stomach, hobbies such as making toy soldiers or stained glass objects, part-time jobs in battery and other lead manufacturing plants, metal working shops, home repair involving burning and scraping of old painted surfaces, use of illicit alcoholic beverages, and biting of lead-dirt laden fingernails). If all ages in a household are involved, suspect a common source (i.e., use of improperly lead-glazed pottery cups and/or pitchers for fruit juice and other acidic beverages, burning of battery casings or old painted boards, collection and storage of drinking water in lead-lined cisterns, and use of contaminated herbal or "health" preparations).

Toxicity: The actual dose of lead absorbed is rarely known. The degree of toxicity, risk of acute symptoms, and need for chelation therapy can be estimated on the basis of certain laboratory tests. Ranges in whole blood lead concentration (μg Pb per 100 ml of whole blood) provide an index of current absorption as well as an index of relative risk of symptoms (need special low lead or low trace metal tubes for lead level): <30 μg Pb (normal); 30 to 49 μg Pb (some increase in absorption and environmental exposure, no risk of central nervous system symptoms, developmental toxicity risk moderate); 50 to 69 μg Pb (increased absorption, subclinical toxicity if metabolic tests are also abnormal, mild symptoms uncommon but may be present, developmental toxicity risk high); >70 μg Pb (if confirmed, greatly increased absorption, severe symptoms may occur, metabolic tests probably are abnormal, chelation therapy is indicated even if symptoms are absent). Long bone x-rays positive for "lead lines" in association with 50 to 60 μg Pb or greater indicate a prolonged (6 months or more), increased intake and the need for intervention. ("Lead lines" are uncommon after 6 years of age due to normal bone density.) Routine blood tests may show findings characteristic of iron-deficiency anemia; however, serum iron and total iron-binding capacity are normal if this anemia is caused by lead alone.

Special Tests for Poisoning: Elevated free erythrocyte protoporphyrin levels reflect adverse effects of lead on hemoglobin synthesis in the bone marrow and usually indicate several months of exposure. Several laboratory methods are used to make the determination so the interpretation of the results may vary (iron-deficiency anemia and protoporphyria may also give elevated levels). Generally, levels greater than 150 μg/100 ml packed red blood cells or 50 μg/100 ml whole blood are considered elevated.

Blood lead levels should be drawn with a stainless steel (no solder) vacutainer needle and low lead or low trace metal vacutainer, if possible. Only the BD Plastipak syringe, BD discarded needle, and Abbott butterfly are known to be suitable alternatives.[1] Urine collections should be directly into specially prepared, heavy, metal-free containers.

Basophilic stippling of the red blood cells (if present) or a strongly positive urinary coproporphyrin suggest lead toxicity.

Special Considerations: The response to lead exposure appears to be influenced by dietary factors. Enhanced absorption, retention, blood lead levels, and toxicity have been noted clinically with a deficient intake of calcium. Enhanced absorption and retention have been shown exper-

---

1. Chisolm, J.J., Jr.: Personal communication.

imentally with a deficient intake of calcium, iron, copper, zinc, and selenium and an excessive dietary intake of fat.

The clinical manifestations of lead poisoning are more severe in the summertime.

Screening of populations at risk (1- to 6-year-old children) is appropriate to identify children with increased body burdens of lead. The source of the lead should be identified so exposure can be interrupted and a medical evaluation of the child should be obtained. Lead appears to cause a developmental disorder characterized by behavioral, educational, and neurologic abnormalities. The development of these abnormalities, now thought to be permanent, can occur in children who have no symptoms or signs which would direct medical attention to the primary cause. Identification of the cause is difficult by the time school problems occur.

Symptoms and Findings: Significant blood lead levels and indications of adverse metabolic effects can be present without overt symptoms.

Infants and Toddlers—Early symptoms (e.g., anorexia, irritability, occasional vomiting, mild stomachaches, refusal to play, and other behavior changes) and findings (e.g., anemia) are nonspecific and are commonly found in other illnesses in this age group. Toddlers with an apparent iron deficiency should also be tested for increased lead absorption. Plumbism in this group frequently is not recognized until an acute encephalopathic state occurs (e.g., persistent vomiting, stupor, ataxia, intractable convulsions, coma). Even at the encephalopathic state, special tests described previously will need to be done to establish the diagnosis, but chelation therapy must be started promptly on the basis of a presumptive diagnosis in any child who is symptomatic.

Older Preschool Children—The clinical presentation described for infants and toddlers is less common in this age group. Instead they may have a nonspecific seizure disorder, developmental regression, autism, or severe behavior disorder.

School Age, Adolescent—Acute poisoning: metallic taste, dry mouth, nausea, vomiting, irritability, weakness, colicky abdominal pain, constipation, pain and tenderness in arms and legs. In severe, acute poisoning, there may be a hemolytic crisis and/or renal injury.

Children with sickle cell disease may be at a greater risk of severe symptomatology from lead exposure. Symptoms may regress spontaneously in all age groups if the excessive intake abates.

Exposure to tetraethyl lead in gasoline from sniffing abuse may produce predominantly cerebellar symptoms and personality changes. In addition to severe central nervous system symptoms, some patients may have peripheral nervous system, muscle, hepatic, and renal damage.

Treatment: The identification of the source of overexposure and separation from it is the most important aspect of treatment. Institution of a balanced diet with adequate calcium, iron, protein, and trace metals is beneficial. Chelation therapy serves to reduce dangerous soft tissue lead levels quickly and is most efficacious if it is given in the subclinical stage on the basis of clearly abnormal metabolic tests.

Acute Symptomatic Plumbism – If the patient has status epilepticus, give diazepam (0.05 to 0.1 mg/kg, slowly intravenously) to obtain initial control of the seizures. Thereafter, use paraldehyde to maintain control (2 to 5 ml in cottonseed oil by rectum). Give doses of anticonvulsants in the prodromal stage, as needed, until the patient is recovered and started on long-term anticonvulsant therapy. Establish an adequate urine flow, but do not overhydrate. Initially, give 10% dextrose and water intravenously (10 to 20 gm/kg) over 1 to 2 hours. If this fails to establish an adequate urine flow, try mannitol (1 to 2 gm/kg, intravenously) in a 20% solution at a rate of 1 ml per minute. After the urine flow is established, restrict the intravenous fluid therapy to basal water and electrolyte requirements and minimal estimate of replacement needs. Adjust the infusion to produce a urine output of 1 ml/kg per 24 hours. Taper the infusion and begin oral liquids only when the symptoms have abated (usually 1 to 4 days). Surgical decompression is contraindicated. Do not waste time with an enema if the patient is symptomatic. Even mildly symptomatic patients, asymptomatic patients with blood lead levels of 100 μg, and patients with abnormal metabolic tests should be treated with precautions. Do not give medicinal iron (oral or parenteral) concurrently with BAL (dimercaprol); use transfusions, if they are absolutely necessary for severe anemia. Chelation therapy: BAL in oil (4 mg/kg per dose) given deep intramuscularly every 4 hours; CaEDTA 20% solution (75 mg/kg per 24 hours) with 0.5 ml of 1% procaine or lidocaine added to each dose, given deep intramuscularly in divided doses every 4 hours. First dose, inject BAL only. Four hours later and every 4 hours thereafter for 5 to 7 days, inject BAL and CaEDTA at separate, rotated, deep intramuscular sites. For encephalopathy, give a full 5- to 7-day course. Repeat courses may be necessary a few days to weeks later. In milder cases without central nervous system symptoms, BAL may be discontinued after 3 days, and CaEDTA may be reduced to 50 mg/kg per 24 hours, divided into two intramuscular doses every 12 hours. Penicillamine (investigational use) has been used for follow-up therapy (20 to 40 mg/kg per day orally) in divided doses on an empty stomach, for no more than a week at a time, but it is not recommended for initial therapy.

Subclinical Plumbism – Some physicians administer CaEDTA (1,000 mg/M^2 per 24 hours in divided doses every 12 hours intramuscularly, for 3 to 5 days) to patients with blood lead levels of 50 to 70 μg and abnormal FEP tests. Penicillamine (investigational use), 500 mg/M^2 per day, given orally as a single dose 2 hours before breakfast, has been used for follow-up therapy. Patients on penicillamine should have urinalysis (proteinuria, red blood cells) and complete blood count with white count and differential (neutropenia) at least weekly. Other physicians consider control of exposure and proper diet more important than drug therapy for patients with subclinical plumbism.

Prospectively Screened Asymptomatic Children with Elevated Blood Lead Levels – Recheck the venous blood lead level because the risk of contamination in collection and errors in analysis are considerable. Obtain a careful environmental history for possible sources. In general, patients with blood lead levels between 50 and 70 μg/100 gm and EP levels >60 μg/100 ml whole blood who have positive long bone x-rays for lead lines or an abnormal EDTA challenge test (0.5 μg Pb excreted in urine in 8 hours for each milligram of EDTA given, or if the ratio of lead in micrograms per liter in 24-hour urine to milligrams of EDTA administered equals 1 or more) should be chelated with EDTA. 1,000 mg/M^2 per day in two divided doses for 5 days. Challenge dose: 1,000 mg/M^2 for 8-hour test or 50 mg CaEDTA per kilogram, intramuscularly, with 0.5 ml of 1% procaine or lidocaine for 24-hour test.

In organic lead poisoning, use of chelation therapy is based on blood lead levels only, not FEP.

References:

Preventing lead poisoning in young children. A statement by the Center for Disease Control. J. Pediat., **93**:709, 1978.

Needleman, H.L., Gunnoe, C., Leviton, A., Reed, R., Peresie, H., Maher, C., and Barrett, P.: Deficits in psychologic and classroom performance of children with elevated dentine lead levels. New Engl. J. Med., **300**:689, 1979.

Mahaffey, K.: Relation between quantities of lead ingested and health effects of lead in humans. Pediatrics, **59**:448, 1977.

Chisolm, J.J., Jr., and Barltrop, D.: Recognition and management of children with increased lead absorption. Arch. Dis. Child., **54**:249, 1979.

Chisolm, J.J., Jr.: Heme metabolites in blood and urine in relation to lead toxicity and their determination. *In* Bodansky, O., and Latner, A.L., ed.: Advances Clinical Chemistry, Vol. 20. New York: Academic Press, p. 225, 1979.

Mahaffey, K.R.: Nutritional factors in lead poisoning. Nutr. Rev., **39**:353, 1981.

Boeckx, R.L., Posti, B., and Coodin, F.J.: Gasoline sniffing and tetraethyl lead poisoning in children. Pediatrics, **60**:140, 1977.

LSD
(Lysergic Acid Diethylamide; Lysergide)

Type of Product: Hallucinogen.

Manufacturer: No legal manufacturer except for research trade.

Ingredients/Description: LSD can be a powder, a tablet, in a sugar cube, a drop evaporated on filter or blotting paper called a "microdot," or in a gelatin square called a "windowpane." Street names: "Acid," "Heavenly Blue," "Pearly Gates," "Flying Saucers," "Wedding Bells," "Summer Skies."

Source: Ergot fungus derivative.

Toxicity: As little as 10 to 20 μg has produced altered mental states; 100 μg is the most common dose used by adults; 100 to 400 μg can be extremely intoxicating.

Symptoms and Findings: LSD has the ability to alter cognitive and perceptual states by its action on the central nervous system. Following recreational ingestion of LSD, changes occur in visual perceptions (such as intensified colors); objects seem to acquire a third dimension and have an emotional impact. Changes also occur in auditory, tactile, and other sensory perceptions. Personality changes can ensue, with the possibility of psychopathic, homicidal and/or suicidal urges, disordered thought processes, alterations in time and space, and severe fluctuations in mood. Dizziness, a feeling of pins and needles, sweating, dilated pupils, restlessness, and acute anxiety can also develop. The sense of body position and placement may be deranged. Skeletal muscle tension, incoordination, and tremors also can develop. LSD can produce nausea, vomiting, and diarrhea as well as hypertension or hypotension.

The effects usually develop within 30 to 90 minutes after ingestion. The acute symptoms may wear off in 5 to 8 hours, and the patient may experience fatigue and tension. "Flashbacks" or psychotic episodes sometimes occur several weeks or months after the exposure. Such flashbacks may produce the same symptoms as the original experience.

Treatment: The establishment or stabilization of respirations may be necessary. Induce emesis (Ipecac Syrup, p. 3). If emesis is contraindicated, perform a gastric lavage with a large-bore tube after an endotracheal tube is in place (p. 4). It is unknown whether or not activated charcoal effectively absorbs LSD, but it does act as a gastrointestinal marker (p. 4). A cathartic (magnesium sulfate or sodium sulfate, 250 mg/kg for a child and 30 gm per/dose for an adult) may help remove any unabsorbed LSD from the gastrointestinal tract. Diazepam (either intravenously or intramuscularly) may be useful in decreasing the anxiety.

References:

Grogan, F.: Treatment of LSD-induced psychosis. Hosp. Formulary Management, 8:24, November, 1973.

Levy, R.M.: Diazepam for L.S.D. intoxication. Lancet, 1:1297, 1971.

Aghajanian, G.K.: LSD and central nervous system transmission. Ann. Rev. Pharmacol., 12:157, 1972.

Shulgin, A.T.: Profiles of psychedelic drugs 9. LSD. J. Psychedelic Drugs, 12:173, 1980.

Klock, J.C., Boerner, U., and Becker, C.E.: Coma, hyperthermia and bleeding associated with massive LSD overdose: A report of eight cases. Western J. Med., 120:183, 1973.

Ianzito, B.M., Liskow, B., and Stewart, M.A.: Reaction to LSD in a two-year-old child. J. Pediat., 80:643, 1972.

Meprobamate

Type of Product: Hypnotic, sedative muscle relaxant, minor tranquilizer.

Manufacturer: Miltown, Meprosan – Wallace; Equanil – Wyeth; and generics.

Ingredients/Description: Meprobamate supplied as: tablets, 200, 400, and 600 mg; coated tablets, 200 and 400 mg; capsules, 400 and 600 mg; liquid, 200 mg/5 ml; 200 and 400 mg sustained-release capsules. Also in combination with other drugs in various dose forms.

Toxicity: Death has been reported in acute overdoses in adults after ingestion of 10 and 12 gm, although survival has occurred after a 40 gm dose. Absorption is usually rapid, but large amounts of meprobamate may form a chemical bezoar in the stomach. This may result in a persistent elevation of plasma levels and prolonged or recurrent coma. Elimination is predominantly by metabolism, although 10% is excreted unchanged. Forced diuresis increases meprobamate clearance, but it should be used cautiously because there appears to be a propensity for pulmonary edema to occur in this overdose.

Symptoms and Findings: Central nervous system depression with lethargy, stupor, ataxia, deep sleep, coma, and shock. Generally, respiration, blood pressure, and pulse parallel the depth of sedation; however, occasional patients have hypotension that does not correlate with coma. Profound shock associated with vasomotor and respiratory collapse may occur. Convulsions have been noted during recovery. Recurrence of a higher degree of coma has occurred and suggests a gastric mass of unabsorbed meprobamate.

Treatment: Induce emesis (Ipecac Syrup, p. 3) or perform gastric lavage (p. 4). After evacuation of the stomach, administer activated charcoal (p. 4) and a saline cathartic (p. 5). Maintain respiration. Correct hypotension with fluids judiciously and vasopressors (levarterenol or metaraminol) cautiously because pulmonary edema or cardiac failure may occur.

Some clinicians advise diuresis with furosemide (1 mg/kg) after rehydration. Carefully monitor fluid input and output. Both charcoal hemoperfusion and hemodialysis remove meprobamate from plasma, but their influence on outcome has not been fully evaluated.

If a gastric mass (bezoar) is suspected, an x-ray of the abdomen with gastric insufflation, instillation of gastrographin, or thin barium may define the presence of unabsorbed drug, or a gastroscopy may be done. Gastrostomy may be necessary for the removal of observed masses.

References:

Maddock, R.K., Jr., and Bloomer, H.A.: Meprobamate overdosage: Evaluation of its severity and methods of treatment. J.A.M.A., 201:999, 1967.

Schwartz, H.S.: Acute meprobamate poisoning with gastrotomy and removal of a drug-containing mass. New Engl. J. Med., 295:1177, 1976.

Gomolin, I.: Meprobamate. Clin. Toxicol., 18:757, No. 6, 1981.

Mercury

Type of Product: Antiseptics, fungicides, pigments, diuretics, ointments, disc batteries, and vapors from elemental form or heating salts.

Ingredients/Description: Many salts of mercury are available as well as elemental mercury and a variety of organomercurials. There is no characteristic form or preparation. They may be as chemicals, pesticides, or medications; and they usually are labelled with the specific mercurial.

Toxicity: The estimated oral fatal dose of mercuric chloride is 0.4 to 4 gm for adults, but fatalities have occurred from 0.2 gm. Poisoning may result from absorption of mercury through the skin from ointments or bichloride of mercury-treated diapers. Small amounts of metallic mercury (as in thermometers) are not toxic on ingestion; however, this type of mercury is difficult to clean up and, when spilled (such as in an infant incubator, bedroom, or laboratory) may slowly vaporize. Inhalation of mercury vapor can cause serious pulmonary illness as well as generalized mercury poisoning. Prolonged contact with disc batteries inside the body may result in serious corrosion as well as systemic poisoning.

Bioaccumulation in the food chain as a result of environmental contamination or the use of contaminated grains for feed has resulted in outbreaks of methylmercury poisoning. In these instances, neurologic manifestations seem to predominate over gastrointestinal and renal manifestations. Conversion of organic to inorganic forms of mercury and vice versa can take place in the body to give mixed symptomatology. The methylmercury bond seems to be the strongest, and it has a prolonged half-life in the body. Phenylmercury rapidly undergoes conversion in the body to an inorganic form. Methylmercury, ethylmercury, and phenylmercury are rapidly absorbed from the gastrointestinal tract.

Inorganic mercury can cross the placental barrier. Organo-mercurials cross the placental barrier even more readily. Methylmercury concentrates in the fetus, even in mothers without symptoms of poisoning; and it concentrates in breast milk at levels lower than in the mother's blood.

Symptoms and Findings: Acute Poisoning—The alimentary absorption of corrosive mercury salts is so rapid that the course and prognosis frequently are determined by the events of the first 15 minutes after ingestion. Early symptoms include violent pain in the upper alimentary tract, profuse vomiting of bloody mucoid material, and severe purging with liquid, bloody stools. These symptoms may progress to prostration, collapse, and death from peripheral vascular collapse.

Mercury vapor inhalation produces a metallic taste, nausea, abdominal pain, vomiting, diarrhea, headache, dyspnea, and occasionally albuminuria. The pulmonary effects may resolve in a few days or progress to necrotizing bronchiolitis, pneumonitis, pulmonary edema, pneumothorax, and death. In milder cases, recovery occurs within 10 to 14 days; in other cases, poisoning of the chronic type accompanied by muscular tremors and psychic disturbances may occur.

By either route of poisoning, in 1 to 3 days the patient may develop swelling of the salivary glands, stomatitis, renal tubular degeneration, and anuria.

Many organic mercurial compounds used in agriculture, especially methylmercury, produce severe central nervous system symptoms, including ataxia, speech and hearing impairment, constriction of visual fields, and delirium. Depending on the type of organomercurial, the patient may develop stomatitis, gastritis, colitis, and renal damage as seen in inorganic mercury poisoning.

Chronic Inorganic Mercury Poisoning — Because mercury is a cumulative poison, the disease may become manifest insidiously. There may be vasomotor disturbances in the skin with inflammatory reactions, eczema, petechial hemorrhages, excessive perspiration, desquamation of the skin, and dystrophy of the fingernails. Gastrointestinal symptoms are characterized by either an increase in or lack of appetite, foul breath, salivation, metallic taste, gingivitis, stomatitis, vomiting, and diarrhea. The gingiva may be spongy and ulcerated, and the teeth may be discolored, fragile, and loose. Nervous system symptoms include irritability, mental hyperactivity, insomnia, anxiety, easy fatigability, slowed mentation, forgetfulness, timidity, loss of memory, and childishness. Neuromuscular disturbances include fine intention tremors starting in the fingers and extending to the arms and legs; jerky movements of the limbs, the head, and the trunk may appear later; there may be a loss of coordination, unsteady gait, exaggerated deep reflexes, and clonus. Death is usually the result of complete renal failure.

Acrodynia (Pink Disease) — Although recognized only rarely today, a symptom complex of irritability, diaphoresis, skin rashes, tachycardia, increased blood pressure, photophobia, anorexia, poor muscle tone (especially of the pectoral and pelvic girdles), red palms and soles, swelling of the hands and feet, and diarrhea or constipation may be associated with chronic mercury exposure in young children. This has occurred from exposure to mercurous chloride contained in teething lotion and diaper powders, mercuric chloride used as a diaper rinse, the heating of paint containing a mercurial for mildew control, and an organic mercurial bacteriostatic agent in repeatedly administered gamma-globulin.

Intra-uterine exposure to inorganic mercury may result in tremors and involuntary movements in the infant. Such exposure to methylmercury resulted in various degrees of motor and mental development with cerebral palsy, deafness, blindness, microcephaly, fretfulness, irritability, and excessive crying.

In all mercury poisonings except methylmercury, properly collected blood and 24-hour urine samples for mercury levels may help in establishing the diagnosis and in following the efficacy and duration of therapy. Methylmercury is minimally excreted in urine; early in the course of exposure or after prolonged exposure, the intensity of the exposure may not be determined by its level in blood.

Diagnostic levels for mercury in blood and urine are not well established, but it appears that levels greater than 2 to 4 μg/dl in blood and 10 to 20 μg/l in urine are above the average of nonoccupationally exposed adults.

Treatment: Immediately induce emesis (Ipecac Syrup, p. 3) or perform a gastric lavage (p. 4). Give egg white or milk. Immediately administer BAL (dimercaprol) by deep intramuscular injection (4 mg/kg), even before attempts to evacuate the stomach. Continue BAL administration (4 mg/kg) every 4 hours for at least 2 days; the dose may then be tapered, depending on the patient's condition and the mercury excretion. Treat shock by correcting dehydration and electrolyte imbalance. Monitor blood gases, electrolytes, and hemoglobin levels. Obtain blood and 24-hour urine mercury levels (consult the laboratory for proper collection technique and containers). Watch for acute renal failure. If instituted early with concurrent BAL administration, peritoneal or hemodialysis may control uremia, give the kidneys a chance to recover, and remove some mercury. Peritoneal dialysis should be used if oliguria or renal shutdown occurs.

N-acetyl-d-L-penicillamine (investigational use) is effective as an oral chelator after the acute phase of mercury poisoning or for acrodynia; 100 mg/kg per 24 hours, up to 1 gm per 24 hours may be given in divided doses orally on an empty stomach 1 hour before meals. Penicillamine also has been used, but it is not as specific a chelator. Monitor 24-hour urine mercury levels to determine when to stop chelation therapy.

In mercury vapor inhalation, pulmonary toxicity should be anticipated, and serial blood gases and chest x-rays should be monitored. Chelation therapy should be instituted promptly because the mercury vapor quickly goes to the brain, where it becomes converted to an inorganic salt. Oxygen and mist therapy may be needed. The administration of prophylactic antibiotics, bronchodilators, and steroids should be considered.

To date, the treatment of subacute and chronic methylmercury poisoning has been of limited effectiveness. Based on animal experiments, BAL seems contraindicated. The oral chelators (experimental) 2, 3 dimercaptosuccinic acid or N-acetyl-d-L-penicillamine and/or interruption of enterohepatic circulation using a polythiol resin (experimental) may be helpful. Limited experience with a regional hemodialyzer system using L-cysteine as a chelating agent is promising.

Other organomercurials should be treated as described for chronic mercury poisoning.

References:

Gosselin, R.E., Hodge, H.C., Smith, R.P., and Gleason, M.N.: Clinical Toxicology of Commercial Products: Acute Poisoning, ed. 4. Baltimore: Williams and Wilkins, Sect. III, pp. 223-229, 1976, reprinted 1977.

Miller, M.W., and Clarkson, T.W.: Mercury, Mercurials, and Mercaptans. Springfield, Illinois: Charles C Thomas, 1973.

Moutinho, M.E., Tompkins, A.L., Rowland, T.W., Banson, B.B., and Jackson, A.H.: Acute mercury vapor poisoning: Fatality in an infant. Amer. J. Dis. Child., 135:42, 1981.

Kark, R.A.P., Poskanzer, D.C., Bullock, J.D., and Boylen, G.: Mercury poisoning and its treatment with N-acetyl-D,L-penicillamine. New Engl. J. Med., 285:10, 1971.

Aronow, R., and Fleischmann, L.E.: Mercury poisoning in children. Clin. Pediat., 15:936, 1976.

Votteler, T.P.: Warning: Ingested disc batteries. Texas Med., 77:7, February, 1981.

Dales, L.G.: The neurotoxicity of alkyl mercury compounds. Amer. J. Med., 53:219, 1972.

Sanchez-Sicilia, L., Seto, D., Nakamoto, S., and Kolff, W.J.: Acute mercurial intoxication treated by hemodialysis. Ann. Intern. Med., 59:692, 1963.

Swaiman, K.F., and Flagler, D.G.: Mercury poisoning with central and peripheral nervous system involvement treated with penicillamine. Pediatrics, 48:639, 1971.

Matheson, D.S., Clarkson, T.W., and Gelfand, E.W.: Mercury toxicity (acrodynia) induced by long-term injection of gammaglobulin. J. Pediat., 97:153, 1980.

Methaqualone

Type of Product: Hypnotic.

Ingredients/Description: 150 mg tablets (QuaaLude-150, Sopor), 200 mg capsules (Parest-200), 300 mg tablets (QuaaLude-300, Mequin, Sopor), 400 mg capsules (Parest-400).

QuaaLude, Mequin, and Sopor contain a methaqualone base. Parest contains methaqualone HCl; 200 mg of methaqualone HCl contains 175 mg of base, and 400 mg of methaqualone HCl contains 350 mg of base.

There are many street sources of methaqualone. Some street "methaqualone" has been found not to contain methaqualone.

Toxicity: In adults, oral doses of 8 to 20 gm (100 to 200 mg/kg) have caused death; survival has followed the ingestion of as much as 24 gm (more than 300 mg/kg). Large amounts of alcohol were also ingested in some fatal cases. Delay in starting supportive care has been a factor in some deaths when doses were in the moderate range. There is a correlation between dose, severity of symptoms, and the duration of sedation.

Symptoms and Findings: With low toxic doses (40 to 80 mg/kg), symptoms are similar to other sedatives; dizziness, ataxia, slurred speech, drowsiness, nystagmus, nausea, vomiting, and epigastric discomfort have been reported. At higher doses, increased muscle tone, agitation, increased motor activity, and tonic convulsions are usually seen. Deep tendon reflexes may be increased.

Respiratory depresssion is exhibited by poor ventilation, although the respiratory rate may be normal or increased. The cough reflex may be dimished. Blood pressure generally is normal. In severe poisoning (>200 mg/kg), deep coma, hypotension, tachycardia, oliguria, hemorrhage (in the gastrointestinal tract, retina, or skin), liver toxicity, respiratory depression, apnea, and cerebral and pulmonary edema have been reported. Up-going plantar reflexes have been reported but are uncommon; deep tendon reflexes and corneal and gag reflexes are absent. Polyneuropathy is reported. Tonic seizures are associated with dysrhythmic pattern on an electroencephlogram. Pupils are middilation and fixed. Both hypothermia and hyperthermia may occur, but the hyperthermia may be a sign of aspiration pneumonia.

Treatment: If the patient is still alert with gag reflex, induce emesis (Ipecac Syrup, p. 3). If the patient is in a coma, perform a gastric lavage with normal saline after a snug-fitting endotracheal tube is in place (p. 4). Supportive measures include assisted ventilation when clinically indi-

cated, maintenance of urinary output, and fluid and electrolyte balance. Forced diuresis has little value. Treat tonic
seizures with diazepam (0.05 to 0.1 mg/kg, intravenously). If
toxicity is severe, succinylcholine with supportive ventilation
may be required. Hemodialysis may be used. Although
dialysance is not high, accelerated clinical improvement has
been reported. Results of peritoneal dialysis have been dis-
appointing. Hemoperfusion may be helpful in severe cases.
Isoproterenol or levarterenol infusions may be used, along
with appropriate hydration with a balanced hydrating fluid
or plasma expanders to elevate the blood pressure.

References:

Ager, S.A.: Luding out. New Engl. J. Med., 287:51, 1972.

Matthew, H., Proudfoot, A.T., Brown, S.S., and Smith, A.C.A.:
Mandrax poisoning: Conservative management of 116 patients.
Brit. Med. J., 2:101, 1968.

Mills, D.G.: Effects of methaqualone on blood platelet function. Clin.
Pharm. Ther., 23:685, 1978.

Abboud, R.T., Freedman, M.T., Rogers, R.M., and Daniele, R.P.:
Methaqualone poisoning with muscular hyperactivity necessitating
the use of curare. Chest, 65:204, 1974.

Majelyne, W., DeClerck, F., Demeter, I., and Heyndrickx, A.:
Treatment evaluation of a severe methaqualone intoxication in man.
Veterin. Human Toxicol., 21:201, 1979.

Methyl Alcohol

Type of Product: Solvent (especially for shellac and paint
remover), nonpermanent-type antifreeze, deicers, window
washer fluid, duplicating fluid, fuel (e.g., model airplane);
often called wood alcohol. Ten percent methanol by volume
is added to gasoline to make gasohol.

Ingredients/Description: Clear fluid with a slight, distinctive
odor.

Toxicity: There is no safe dose. Although rare, poisoning can
occur through skin absorption or by inhalation. One tea-
spoonful of methanol ingested is potentially lethal for a
2-year-old child and can cause blindness in an adult. Two
to 8 oz (1 ml/kg) may be lethal for an adult. Manifestations
of toxicity are mainly related to the metabolic products of

methyl alcohol: formic acid and formaldehyde. Methyl alcohol is metabolized (at one-fifth to one-ninth the rate of ethanol) in the liver through alcohol dehydrogenase utilizing NAD. This substrate may become depleted and gluconeogenesis may become impaired, with resulting hypoglycemia. A small percentage of a dose of methanol is excreted unchanged by the kidneys and through respiration. The accumulation of formic acid plus a possible cellular block in energy metabolism leads to a profound acidosis; it may also account for optic nerve damage.

Ethanol is bound more tightly to metabolic sites than methanol. When ingested together, ethanol is nearly completely eliminated before methanol is metabolized. In combination with ethanol, the methanol toxicity may be delayed.

Symptoms and Findings: Initially the patient may be symptom free or inebriated and drowsy, and there may be a delay of development of severe acidosis and visual disturbances for 12 to 48 hours. There may be dysphoria; nausea; vomiting; abdominal pain; weakness; dilated, unreactive pupils and dimness of vision; hyperpnea; cyanosis; delirium; convulsions; and coma. Blood chemistries may reveal severe metabolic acidosis, a large anion gap, and an increased freezing-point depression measured osmolarity over calculated osmolarity. Cerebral edema may develop. Death is caused by respiratory failure or circulatory collapse. Permanent loss of vision may occur in survivors. Blood methyl alcohol levels do not correlate with visual disturbances or their outcome. Prompt and energetic therapy must be initiated. Do not wait for the development of symptoms. Pancreatitis also has been found in some lethal cases. Institute supportive and symptomatic care.

Treatment: For all patients, empty the stomach, regardless of the amount ingested, either by inducing emesis (Ipecac Syrup, p. 3) or performing a gastric lavage (see p. 4). Determine the blood methanol level. Obtain electrolyte, glucose, and arterial blood gas measurements. Administer maintenance fluids. Treat acidosis vigorously with sodium bicarbonate intravenously (3 to 5 mEq/kg) to restore normal blood pH. Initiate ethanol therapy (see p. 15); the route depends on the patient's clinical status. The goal is to create a blood ethanol level of 100 to 150 mg% (mg/dl) to saturate alcohol dehydrogenase in the liver and prevent further metabolism of the methyl alcohol. The loading dose of ethanol is approximately 1 to 1½ ml of 100% alcohol (0.79 gm) per kilogram; the maintenance dose is based on the calculated rate of metabolism of ethanol (approximately 125 mg/kg per hour). If it is given intravenously, ethanol should be diluted to 5 to 10%, usually in D_5W. Ethanol blood levels must be monitored, and ethanol administration must be continued for at least 24 hours after the acidosis is corrected or the methanol is cleared from the body. No more than 10% of methanol is excreted through the urine; so, if a serious poisoning exists, dialysis must be used to clear the methanol from the body. Hemodialysis is much more effective in clearing methanol than peritoneal dialysis and should be instituted if the blood methanol level is 50 mg/dl or more or if the symptoms progress rapidly. Dialysis will necessitate increasing the ethanol dose a variable amount, depending on the efficiency of the dialysis system[1] (p. 16).

Methanol is an eye irritant, and irrigation (p. 6) should be undertaken for at least 15 minutes if it has gotten into an eye.

References:

Gosselin, R.E., Hodge, H.C., Smith, R.P., and Gleason, M.N.: Clinical Toxicology of Commercial Products, ed. 4. Baltimore: Williams and Wilkins, Section III, pp. 229-233, 1976, reprinted 1977.

Kahn, A., and Blum, D.: Methyl alcohol poisoning in an 8-month-old boy: An unusual route of intoxication. J. Pediat., 94:841, 1979.

McMartin, K.E., Ambre, J.J., and Tephly, T.R.: Methanol poisoning in human subjects: Role for formic acid accumulation in the metabolic acidosis. Amer. J. Med., 68:414, 1980.

Gonda, A., Gault, H., Churchill, D., and Hollomby, D.: Hemodialysis for methanol intoxication. Amer. J. Med., 64:749, 1978.

Tintinalli, J.E.: Of anions, osmols, and methanol poisoning. J. Amer. Coll. Emerg. Phys., 6:417, 1977.

Methyprylon (Noludar)

Type of Product: Nonbarbiturate hypnotic.

---

1. McCoy, H.G., Cipolle, R.J., Ehlers, S.M., Sawchuk, R.J., and Zaske, D.E.: Severe methanol poisoning. Application of a pharmacokinetic model for ethanol therapy and hemodialysis. Amer. J. Med., 67:804, 1979.

Manufacturer: Roche Laboratories, Division Hoffman-La Roche Inc.

Ingredients/Description: Methyprylon, 50 mg and 200 mg tablets; 300 mg capsules.

Toxicity: A 64-year-old adult died after ingesting 6.0 gm. Others have survived 30.0 gm with supportive care only. Although the drug itself causes symptoms, slow recovery with poor return of the drug after dialysis has been attributed to toxic metabolites. No direct evidence for such metabolites has been presented. The half-life of therapeutic doses of the drug is 4 to 6 hours.

Symptoms and Findings: Nausea, vomiting, diarrhea, drowsiness, ataxia, excitation, convulsions, coma, hyperpyrexia or hypopyrexia, shallow respiration, small pupils, or hypotension may be present.

Treatment: Induce emesis (Ipecac Syrup, p. 3) or perform gastric lavage (p. 4). Administer activated charcoal (p. 4) and a saline laxative (p. 5).
Prevent hypoxia by use of intubation, respiratory support, and oxygen as needed. Use intravenous fluids as indicated by renal output, blood pressure, and central venous pressure. Hypotension may require vasopressors (dopamine or metaraminol). Peritoneal dialysis and hemodialysis have been effective in limited, reported cases. Charcoal hemoperfusion may be used, although the efficacy of this therapy has not been great and the need for its use is not clear.

References:

Polin, R.A., Henry, D., and Pippinger, C.E.: Peritoneal dialysis for severe methyprylon intoxication. J. Pediat., **90**:831, 1977.
Pancorbo, A.S., Palagi, P.A., Piecoro, J.J., and Wilson, H.D.: Hemodialysis in methyprylon overdose: Some pharmacokinetic considerations. J.A.M.A., **237**:470, 1977.

Multivitamin Preparations

Type of Product: Dietary supplement.

Ingredients/Description: Vary with the product and manufacturer.

Toxicity: There is little toxicity from acute ingestions, and it relates primarily to iron and the fat-soluble vitamins A and D. See Iron Salts (p. 75) for a full discussion of iron toxicity and therapy.

Single ingestions of vitamin A of 75,000 to 300,000 IU in infants and at least 2,000,000 IU in adults may cause toxicity within a few hours. A decision on excess ingestion may be aided by a serum level if available. The normal blood level of vitamin A is about 30 to 70 μg/100 ml. The prolonged daily intake of 7,000 to 10,000 IU of vitamin A over the Recommended Daily Allowance may cause toxic symptoms. Increased intracranial pressure is the most common feature of both acute and chronic vitamin A intoxication.

Vitamin D is stored in the body and not readily excreted. Sensitivity to vitamin D varies among individuals, with a narrow margin of safety between therapeutic and toxic doses in infants and children. Most symptoms of hypervitaminosis D are the result of deranged calcium metabolism. No vitamin D single, toxic-dose level has been established. In chronic exposure, symptoms of toxicity may occur with doses of 1,000 IU or more daily, and retardation of linear growth has been reported with doses of 1,800 IU daily. As little as 50,000 IU's per day over a month has produced toxicity in adults, whereas much larger doses have been tolerated for prolonged periods.

Symptoms and Findings: In acute vitamin A overdose in infants, buldging fontanelles, hyperirritability, anorexia, and vomiting may occur. In chronic overdose (a few months), pseudotumor cerebri (intracranial hypertension), widening of sutures with buldging fontanelles, increased cerebrospinal fluid pressure, lethargy, tinnitus, pruritis, exfoliative dermatitis, angular stomatitis, hyperostoses, metaphyseal cupping and thickening, paronychia, papilledema, and even optic atrophy may occur.

In adults, acute vitamin A overdose may cause dizziness, severe headache, nausea, vomiting, drowsiness, and erythema which may eventually peel. Hypervitaminosis A in adults (may require years) most commonly causes vomiting, skin changes, irritability, headache, hypomenorrhea, and weakness. Psychiatric symptoms and hepatic dysfunction have also been reported. Most symptoms disappear when the vitamin is discontinued, but premature epiphyseal closure and retardation of growth may occur in children.

Early symptoms of hypervitaminosis D may be vomiting,

anorexia, irritability, polyuria, polydipsia, diarrhea, and headache; these symptoms may later be followed by weakness, fatigue, decreased renal function and hypercalcemia, soft tissue calcifications, irreversible renal failure, and possibly death. Prolonged hypervitaminosis D in infants may result in mental and physical retardation.

Treatment: Induce emesis (Ipecac Syrup, p. 3) or perform gastric lavage (p. 4), followed by activated charcoal (p. 4) and a saline cathartic (p. 5). (If children's chewable multiple vitamin preparations are ingested, a laxative may be eliminated as the fillers and sugars in the vitamin pills tend to act as a laxative.)

In hypervitaminosis A, increased intracranial pressure can be treated with dexamethasone, 4 mg immediately and 1 mg every 4 to 6 hours for infants and children. Alternately, mannitol can be used intravenously in a dose of 1 gm/kg, intravenously, to a maximum of 25 gm per dose. Blood pressure and fluid balance monitoring is mandatory.

Generally, treatment for hypervitaminosis D consists of withdrawal of the vitamin, a low-calcium diet, administration of steroids, and lots of fluids.

References:

Goodman, A.G., and Gilman, L.S., and Gilman, A.: The Pharmacological Basis of Therapeutics, ed. 6. New York: Macmillan Publishing Company, Inc., 1980.

AMA Drug Evaluations, ed. 4. Chicago: Department of Drugs, American Medical Association, 1980.

Gosselin, R.E., Hodge, H.C., Smith, R.P. and Gleason, M.N.: Clinical Toxicology of Commercial Products, ed. 4. Baltimore: Williams and Wilkins, Sect. II, pp. 172-173, 1976, reprinted 1977.

Pasquariello, P.S., Schut, L., and Borns, P.: Benign increased intracranial hypertension due to chronic vitamin A overdosage in a 26-month-old child. Clin. Pediat., 16:379, 1977.

Lippe, B., Hensen, L., Mendoza, G., Finerman, M., and Welch, M.: Chronic vitamin A intoxication. Amer. J. Dis. Child., 135:634, 1981.

Muenter, M.D., Perry, H.O., and Ludwig, J.: Chronic vitamin A intoxication in adults: Hepatic, neurologic and dermatologic complications. Amer. J. Med., 50:129, 1971.

Davies, M., and Adams, P.H.: The continuing risk of vitamin-D intoxication. Lancet, 2:621, 1978.

Paterson, C.R.: Vitamin-D poisoning: Survey of causes in 21 patients with hypercalcaemia. Lancet, 1:1164, 1980.

Verner, J.V., Jr., Engel, F.L., and McPherson, H.T.: Vitamin D intoxication: A report of 2 cases treated with cortisone. Ann. Intern. Med., 48:765, 1958.

Naphthalene

Type of Product: Moth balls and flakes, toilet bowl deodorizers.

Ingredients/Description: Naphthalene ($C_{10}H_8$) is a colorless, crystalline hydrocarbon from coal tar distillates used in moth balls (now more commonly made with para-dichlorobenezene) and toilet deodorizers and as raw material for aniline dyes (do not confuse naphthalene with the naphthene which is used in the petroleum industry for the cyclic hydrocarbons, C_nH_{2n}, found particularly in the aromatic fractions of petroleum such as kerosene).

Toxicity: The lethal oral dose of naphthalene is probably 5 to 15 gm, but sensitivity varies considerably. Naphthalene induces hemolytic crisis (after a 1- to 3-day delay) in G-6-PD-deficient individuals and to a lesser degree in normal infants.

Symptoms and Findings: Acute gastrointestinal irritation; central nervous system irritation with headache, sweating, listlessness, confusion, convulsions, coma; irritation of the urinary bladder with dysuria and passage of brown urine (naphthalene derivates); acute intravascular hemolysis (primarily in G-6-PD-deficient patients) by day 3, with anemia, jaundice, and hemoglobinuria.

Of the symptoms reported, only the gastrointestinal pain seems clearly linked to direct naphthalene toxicity. The central nervous system signs and symptoms reported may largely be the result of hypoxia secondary to hemolysis. Thus, early symptoms are not correlated with severity of toxicity, which is the result of the hematologic abnormality. Attention must be directed toward the prediction, monitoring, and therapy of hemolysis.

Treatment: Induce emesis (Ipecac Syrup, p. 3) or perform gastric lavage (p. 4), followed by activated charcoal and a saline cathartic (p. 5). Do not give mineral or other oils, milk, fatty foods, or alcohol because these substances increase absorption. An immediate screen for the erythrocyte G-6-PD activity, reticulocytosis, methemoglobin, and red cell fragmentation is helpful. If acute hemolytic anemia occurs, treat with hydration, alkaline diuresis, and small transfusions of packed cells.

References:

Gosselin, R.E., Hodge, H.C., Smith, R.P., and Gleason, M.N.: Clinical Toxicology of Commercial Products: Acute Poisoning, ed. 4. Baltimore: Williams and Wilkins, Sect. III, pp. 242-246, 1976, reprinted 1977.

Gidron, E., and Leurer, J.: Naphthalene poisoning. Lancet, 1:228, 1956.

Zuelzer, W.W., and Apt, L.: Acute hemolytic anemia due to naphthalene poisoning: Clinical and experimental study. J.A.M.A., 141:185, 1949.

Valaes, T., Doxiadis, S.A., and Fessas, P.: Acute hemolysis due to naphthalene inhalation. J. Pediat., 63:904, 1963.

Narcotic Analgesics

Type of Product: Analgesic and antidiarrheal agents, including: meperidine (Demerol), methadone (Dolophine), codeine, diphenoxylate (Lomotil), oxycodone (Percodan), pentazocine (Talwin), and morphine, heroin, and opium. For propoxyphene, a related product, see Darvon (p. 57).

Ingredients/Description: Meperidine: Available in tablets of 50 and 100 mg; elixir in bottles of 480 ml which contain 50 mg/50 ml; and vials and ampules for injection containing 25, 50, 75, and 100 mg/ml.

Methadone: Available as injectable with 10 mg/ml or as tablets of 5 mg or 10 mg. Also, effervescent tablets with 2.5, 5, 10, and 40 mg.

Codeine: Various; see the *Physicians' Desk Reference*.

Oxycodone: Available in tablets of 5 mg (yellow) and 2.5 mg (pink), both containing 225 mg aspirin and 32 mg caffeine. Capsules (red), 5 mg, containing 500 mg acetaminophen.

Morphine: Available for injection with 8, 10, and 15 mg/ml.

Opium: Extract of opium is marketed as paregoric with 15 mg opium per ounce.

Lomotil: A combination tablet containing diphenoxylate HCl 2.5 mg and atropine 0.025 mg.

Pentazocine: Available as tablets, 50 mg with 0.5 mg naloxone hydrochloride, and an injectable containing 30 mg/ml in 1.0, 1.5, 2.0, and 10 ml units.

Toxicity: For all narcotics, respiratory depression is the major toxicity leading to death. Doses higher than those recommended therapeutically should be suspect for requiring ventilatory assistance and antidotal therapy. Doses of 75 mg meperidine, 10 mg methadone, 10 mg morphine, and 12.5 mg diphenoxylate have caused serious respiratory depression in children.

Lomotil contains atropine, and early symptoms may be dominated by atropine effects. These symptoms are usually shorter lived than the narcotic effects.

Symptoms and Findings: Respiratory depression is the dominant symptom and cause of death. Other symptoms are divided as:

Central Nervous System: Euphoria, dysphoria, weakness, headache, agitation, nausea, vomiting, uncoordinated muscle movements, hallucinations, disorientation, mental depression, stupor, and coma may occur.

Gastrointestinal: Dry mouth, constipation, and biliary tract spasm with colicky pain may be present.

Cardiovascular: Flushing of the face, tachycardia, bradycardia, palpitation, syncope, circulatory collapse, and cardiac arrest may occur.

Genitourinary: Urinary retention may be found.

Eyes: Pin-point pupils (uncommon with meperidine) may be observed.

Allergic: Itching and urticaria may be present.

Hyperglycemia may be present in narcotic-overdosed children.

After Lomotil ingestion, the symptoms of atropine overdose include flushing, tachycardia, dry mouth, elevated temperature, and agitation (see Atropine, p. 39).

Treatment: Support respiration if its rate or depth has become too low to maintain effective ventilation or if breathing has stopped. If there is no respiratory or central nervous system depression, induce emesis (Ipecac Syrup, p. 3) or perform a gastric lavage (p. 4). Decontaminate the lower gastrointestinal tract. After evacuation of the stomach, administer activated charcoal (p. 4) and a saline cathartic (p. 5).

Naloxone hydrochloride (0.01 mg/kg, intravenously) is the specific antidote. The dose may be safely repeated every 5 to 15 minutes and increased as needed if respirations are not adequate. If three injections produce no significant effect, the diagnosis of narcotic overdose may be in error. Put the patient on an apnea monitor and closely observe. The antidotal action of the narcotic antagonist is shorter than the action of many narcotics, and respiratory depression may recur. Hyperglycemia spontaneously resolves with the administration of the narcotic antagonist. Dialysis is not indicated.

References:

Gosselin, R.E., Hodge, H.C., Smith, R.P., and Gleason, M.N.: Clinical Toxicology of Commercial Products, ed. 4. Baltimore: Williams and Wilkins, Sect. III, pp. 237-242, 1976, reprinted 1977.

Smialek, J.E., Montforte, J.R., Aronow, R., and Spitz, W.U.: Methadone deaths in children: A continuing problem. J.A.M.A., 238:2516, 1977.

Rumack, B.H., and Temple, A.R.: Lomotil poisoning. Pediatrics, 53:495, 1974.

Snyder, R., Mofenson, H.C., and Greensher, J.: Toxicity from Lomotil. Clin. Pediat., 12:47, 1973.

Organochlorine Insecticides

Type of Product: Pesticide.

Ingredients/Description: Organochlorine insecticides are still available in the United States, although they are no longer used as frequently because of their long-range environmental effects. Organochlorine insecticides range from the relatively nontoxic DDT to the highly toxic endrin. Common compounds include chlordane, endrin, dieldrin, lindane, and many others. These compounds are available in liquid, spray, powder, and granular forms. Lindane (benzene hexachloride) is used as a drug (Kwell) for human insect infestation.

Toxicity: These compounds can be absorbed in variable amounts from dermal, respiratory, and oral routes of exposure and are of variable toxicity. They tend to accumulate in man, with the highest concentration being in adipose tissue. The rates of metabolism and excretion vary between compounds and influence the degree of storage. The half-life of a substance may be days in the body from an acute exposure. These compounds primarily stimulate the central nervous system, which results in a sudden onset of convulsions and abnormal functioning of the thermal regulatory apparatus. The exact mechanism of this action is unknown. Stimulation of the hepatic microsome system may also occur. On chronic exposure to chlorinated hydrocarbon pesticides, degenerative changes in the liver and kidney may occur.

Symptoms and Findings: Symptoms may include nausea and vomiting soon after ingestion, although this may be partly caused by the hydrocarbon vehicle frequently used in liquid preparations. Later symptoms and signs are largely related to the nervous system, such as apprehension, paresthesia, excitability, tremor, and muscle twitching. Convulsions are common and may be the first recognized abnormality. Fever, if manifest, will develop after the convulsion. Respiratory depression and coma may ensue. Death may occur rapidly without respiratory support. Lindane is absorbed from the skin, and overuse has resulted in convulsions or erythropoietic hypoplasia.

Treatment: Prevent hypoxia by use of intubation, respiratory support, and oxygen as needed. If the patient is alert, induce emesis (Ipecac Syrup, p. 3). If respirations are depressed, perform a gastric lavage (p. 4). Administer activated charcoal (p. 4).

Wearing gloves, decontaminate the skin and immediately remove soiled garments. Wash the skin carefully (p. 6).

Control convulsions with diazepam (0.05 to 0.1 mg/kg, slowly intravenously) or phenobarbital (5 mg/kg, slowly intravenously). These doses may need to be repeated.

Avoid epinephrine because organochlorine compounds may cause increased myocardial irritability, and epinephrine may induce a life-threatening arrhythmia.

Check for hydrocarbon pneumonitis as the organochlorine may be in a petroleum distillate (p. 84).

References:

Morgan, D.P.: Recognition and Management of Pesticide Poisoning, ed. 3. Washington, D.C.: U.S. Environmental Protection Agency, Office of Pesticide Programs, pp. 14-18, 1982.

Ginsburg, C.M., Lowry, W., and Reisch, J.S.: Absorption of lindane (gamma benzene hexachloride) in infants and children. J. Pediat., 91:998, 1977.
Solomon, L.M., Fahrner, L., and West, D.P.: Gamma benzene hexachloride toxicity: A review. Arch. Dermatol., 113:353, 1977.
Hayes, W.J., Jr.: Pesticides Studied in Man. Baltimore: Williams and Wilkins, pp. 172-283, 1982.

Organophosphate and Carbamate Insecticides

Type of Product: Pesticides in liquid, powder, and granular forms.

Toxicity: Most of these products are absorbed through the skin, gastrointestinal tract, or inhalation and lead to toxicity. The respiratory route of absorption usually leads to a more rapid onset of symptoms. The level of toxicity varies widely from mildly toxic malathion, an organophosphate, and sevin, a carbamate, to parathion and carbaryl, which are highly toxic.

Substances in both groups of compounds bind to acetylcholinesterases, resulting in the build-up of excessive acetylcholine. This leads to all acute symptoms. Organophosphates are released slowly from this enzymatic site; carbamates are released in hours to a day. Acetylcholinesterase regenerators, such as pralidoxime, are helpful with organophosphates; but they are not required with carbamates, and some reports suggest they are harmful with certain carbamates by lengthening the pesticides' residence on the enzymatic site.

Symptoms and Findings: The signs and symptoms may be classified according to three points of action of acetylcholine. The sequence of events outlined here represents a typical course, but variation in the sequence of onset or relative severity of these symptoms between compounds is considerable.

Muscarinic Effects (Parasympathetic Effects) – These symptoms are usually the first to appear and include anorexia, nausea, sweating, epigastric and substernal tightness, heartburn, and tightness in the chest. More severe exposures produce abdominal cramps, increased peristalsis, diarrhea, salivation, lacrimation, profuse sweating, pallor, and dyspnea. Involuntary defecation and urination, excessive bronchial secretions, bronchospasm, and pulmonary edema may occur in severe cases of poisoning.

Nicotinic Effects (Effects on Voluntary Muscles) – These symptoms generally appear after parasympathetic effects have reached moderate severity and include muscle twitching, fasciculations, and cramps, followed by weakness, ataxia, and paralysis.

Central Nervous System Effects – These symptoms are less common than the parasympathetic and muscular effects and may be entirely absent. Symptoms include tension, restlessness, and emotional lability. Greater exposures to organic phosphates produce headaches, tremor, drowsiness, and confusion. Lethal or near lethal doses may produce convulsions, areflexia, coma, and respiratory arrest.

Treatment: Support respiration and overcome cyanosis. Give atropine, 0.05 mg/kg, intravenously, for children and 2 mg for adults, as a starting dose. This dose may be repeated at 5- to 10-minute intervals until all secretions are dry. (Pupils may not dilate with atropine therapy, and this effect should not be used as an end point.) Large total doses of atropine may be required.

If the insecticide was an organophosphate, pralidoxime (2-PAM) should be given intravenously (0.25 gm in children and 1 gm in adults) after atropinization has been achieved; 2-PAM must be given in the first 24 hours for effect. It is not required for all patients, such as those with no significant muscle weakness.

Induce emesis (Ipecac Syrup, p. 3) or perform gastric lavage (p. 4) followed by administration of activated charcoal (p. 4) and a saline laxative (p. 5). Wearing gloves, decontamination of the skin should be performed with Tincture of Green Soap or liquid soap mixed with alcohol to remove the pesticide and oily vehicles. Special attention should be given to washing in skin creases, around the ears, in the external auditory canals, around the umbilicus and genitalia, and under the nails (p. 6).

Red blood cell cholinesterase levels are usually more than 50% depressed for severe symptoms to occur in organophosphate poisonings. If depression is less than 50%, measures should be taken to assure that no futher environmental exposure occurs for 2 to 3 months; this may require assistance from a public health agency in environmental decontamination procedures.

References:

Morgan, D.P.: Recognition and management of pesticide poisonings, ed. 3. Washington, D.C.: U.S. Environmental Protection Agency, Office of Pesticide Programs, pp. 1-13, 1982.
Hayes, W.J., Jr.: Pesticides Studied in Man. Baltimore: Williams and Wilkins, pp. 284-462, 1982.

Paradichlorobenzene

Type of Product: Moth balls and flakes, toilet and diaper pail deodorizer cakes, insecticide.

Ingredients/Description: Paradichlorobenzene is used for killing moths and their larvae, roaches, termites, tree borers, and other insects. It also is used as toilet bowel deodorant cakes, usually with an added perfume of similar volatility. It is commonly found in moth balls and flakes; naphthalene was used more commonly in the past. The two compounds may sometimes be combined.

Toxicity: The lethal oral dose is estimated to be from 500 to 5,000 mg/kg. An ingestion of 20 gm (300 mg/kg) has been well tolerated. Skin absorption is insignificant. Vapors are irritating, and chronic exposure has been reported to result in cataracts or hepatic dysfunction.

Symptoms and Findings: Vapors are irritating to the eyes and mucous membranes, and chronic exposure to them produces headache, vertigo, weakness, and excitement similar to alcohol intoxication. Ingestion of large amounts produces gastrointestinal irritation, pain, nausea, vomiting, and diarrhea. No serious poisonings from ingestion have been reported.

Treatment: Do not give milk, oils, or fatty meals (these increase absorption). Induce emesis (Ipecac Syrup, p. 3) or perform gastric lavage (p. 4). Provide symptomatic and supportive care. Flush the eyes thoroughly with water.

Reference:

Gosselin, R.E., Hodge, H.C., Smith, R.P., and Gleason, M.N.: Clinical Toxicology of Commercial Products: Acute Poisoning, ed.

4. Baltimore: Williams and Wilkins, Sect. II, p. 115, 1976, reprinted 1977.

Phencyclidine (PCP)

Type of Product: Dissociative anesthetic, "drug" of abuse.

Manufacturer: No legitimate manufacturer; "street" sources only.

Ingredients/Description: Phencyclidine (PCP) is now one of the most frequently used ingredients of "street drug" preparations. It is a basic, highly lipid-soluble drug with a pKa between 8.6 and 9.5 that is well absorbed after ingestion, inhalation, or parenteral administration. PCP is strictly a drug of abuse; it no longer is used medically in humans or in veterinary medicine. Abusers refer to it as "PCP," "Angel Dust," "Mist," "Hog," "Crystal," "Rocket Fuel," "Peace Pill," and "Horse Tranquilizer." It is also commonly found in street drugs sold as THC, LSD, psilocybin, and mescaline. More than 38 analogues with similar pharmacologic effects have been identified, including one that contains cyanide. The two most frequently encountered analogues are PCE and PCC. Since 1980, similar products made from a pyrrolidine instead of a piperidine base have been increasingly encountered and are referred to as PHP.

Toxicity: Phencyclidine acts primarily on the central nervous system, either by stimulation or depression. The pharmacologic action in animals and man is complex. The variability in activity makes it difficult to diagnose. The effects of PCP are highly dose dependent in a single exposure, but they may vary in a chronic user and in association with other abused substances. Doses between 0.5 and 1.0 mg/kg of body weight have produced severe agitation, muscle rigidity, and generalized seizure activity. Small children seem particularly susceptible to its anesthetic properties. Laboratory drug screen tests are generally not sensitive enough to pick up doses of PCP that may only alter behavior, nor will they pick up any of the analogues or PHP.

Symptoms and Findings: Common symptoms are excitation or severe paranoid behavior which is frequently self-destructive. However, some patients may be catatonic or have alternating catatony and excitation. Diagnostic clues include: horizontal and vertical nystagmus, tachycardia, hyperhidrosis and salivation, hypertension, seizures, increased reflexes, muscle rigidity, coma, and, with large doses, respiratory depression.

Treatment: Primary efforts should be directed toward managing potentially lethal complications: respiratory and cardiac arrest, status epilepticus, hyperpyrexia, myoglobinuria, and hypertensive crisis. It may be necessary to protect the patient from harm to himself and others. This should include an environment with low sensory input. Exacerbation of clinical symptoms is seen even with minimal verbal or physical stimulation. Care must be taken not to use four extremity restraints because they may exacerbate rhabdomyolysis. Haloperidol (2 to 5 mg intramuscularly, hourly in adults) has been effective for treating behavioral problems. The blood should be monitored for CPK, and the urine should be monitored for the presence of myoglobin.

Gastric lavage with a large-bore gastric tube should be performed followed by administration of activated charcoal (p. 4) and a saline cathartic (p. 5). Excessive muscle activity and seizures should be treated symptomatically with diazepam (child: 0.1 to 0.3 mg/kg, slowly intravenously; adult: 2.5 to 5 mg, slowly intravenously, repeat if needed). Dystonic reactions have been successfully treated with diphenhydramine. The patient's core temperature should be monitored, and hyperthermia should be treated by external cooling measures. Interruption of gastroenteric recycling of the drug may be accomplished by initial continuous gastric drainage or administration of activated charcoal every 6 hours.

Acid diuresis may be of value in ion trapping the phencyclidine. Theoretically, with an alkaline pKa, the PCP should be trapped and excretion enhanced in an acid urine. Some investigators have shown an enhanced excretion of PCP in urine with a pH less than 5.5. When the urine pH is less than 5.5, a diuretic such as furosemide doubles the PCP clearance. No analyses of the metabolic products of PCP have been done, but a dramatic clinical improvement has been reported in life-threatened patients treated in the foregoing manner. Ammonium chloride, orally and/or intravenously, or hydrochloric acid, intravenously, have been used to create an acid urine. Patients who are not life threatened and able to take oral fluids may be given cranberry juice every 6 hours (this juice is metabolized to hippuric acid) to maintain an acid urine.

A careful evaluation of the PCP-overdosed patient for concurrent injuries is important. The lowering of blood pH is contraindicated in closed head injuries, the use of ammonium chloride is contraindicated in liver dysfunction, and acidification of urine is contraindicated in myoglobinuria.

As soon as possible, a psychiatric consultation should be obtained for all except young PCP-overdosed patients. A suspected abuse report should be filed and a social service consultation obtained when young children or infants are exposed to PCP.

References:

Burns, R.S., Lerner, S.E., Corrado, R., James, S.H., and Schnoll, S.H.: Phencyclidine—States of acute intoxication and fatalities. Western J. Med., 123:345, 1975.

Sidoff, M.L.: Phencyclidine: Syndromes of abuse and modes of treatment. Topics Emerg. Med., 1:111, 1979.

Budd, R.D.: PHP, a new drug of abuse. New Engl. J. Med., 303:588, 1980.

Done, A.K., Aronow, R., and Miceli, J.N.: Pharmacokinetic bases for the diagnosis and treatment of acute PCP intoxication. J. Psych. Drugs, 12:253, 1980.

Aronow, R., Miceli, J.N., and Done, A.K.: A therapeutic approach to the acutely overdosed PCP patient. J. Psych. Drugs, 12:259, 1980.

McCarron, M.M., Schulze, B.W., Thompson, G.A., Conder, M.C., and Goetz, W.A.: Acute phencyclidine intoxication: Clinical patterns, complications, and treatment. Ann. Emerg. Med., 10:290, 1981.

Welch, M.J., and Correa, G.A.: PCP intoxication in young children and infants. Clin. Pediat., 19:510, 1980.

Perez-Reyes, M., DiGuiseppi, S., Brine, D.R., Smith, H., and Cook, C.E.: Urine pH and phencyclidine excretion. Clin. Pharm. Therap., 32:635, 1982.

Phenothiazines

Type of Product: Tranquilizer, antiemetic.

Ingredients/Description: The variety of phenothiazine drugs include: (1) aliphatic compounds: chlorpromazine (Thorazine,

Promapar, Chloramead, Foypromazine, Clorazine, Ormazine, Promaz, Psychozine), promazine (Sparine, Norazine, Prozine), triflupromazine (Vesprin); (2) piperidine compounds: thioridazine (Mellaril), piperacetazine (Quide), mesoridazine (Serentil); (3) piperazine compounds: acetophenazine (Tindal), perphenazine (Trilafon), carphenazine (Proketazine), prochlorperazine (Compazine), fluphenazine (Prolixin), trifluoperazine (Stelazine). Other chemically related compounds are: (1) thioxanthene compounds: chlorprothixene (Taractan), thiothixene (Navane); (2) butyrophenone compounds: haloperidol (Haldol); (3) dihydroindolone compounds: molindone (Moban); and (4) dibenzoxazepine compounds: loxapine (Loxitane).

Toxicity: The toxic dose of the phenothiazines has not been well established. Phenothiazines may potentiate central nervous system depressant drugs. Toxicity may be prolonged with sustained-release preparations. Extrapyramidal (Parkinsonian) symptoms may occur with a relatively small overdose of phenothiazine. Infants and children are particularly sensitive to the phenothiazines, as are patients who are toxic, dehydrated, or febrile. Chlorpromazine may have been lethal at oral doses as low as 350 mg in a 4-year-old child and 2 gm in an adult female; a 17-year-old boy survived 17.5 gm. Promazine caused death in a 2-year-old child who ingested 1,000 mg. Fluphenazine ingestions of 20 to 30 mg have been reported in adults without symptoms, and ingestions of unknown amounts caused convulsions and coma. Prochlorperazine caused dysphagia and convulsions in a 4-year-old child after ingesting 30 mg; a 7-year-old child exhibited opisthotonus after a rectal administration of 50 mg.

Phenothiazine-containing drugs are mostly protein bound in the body, with less than 1% eliminated unchanged in the urine.

Symptoms and Findings: Extrapyramidal dyskinetic reactions (such as spasmodic torticollis, oculogyric crisis, akathisia or motor restlessness, jerky movements or twitching of the extremities, hyperirritability, tremors, dysphagia, and other Parkinsonian manifestations) may occur, even after relatively small overdoses. Significant anticholinergic alpha-adrenergic blocking and quinidine-like effects may be seen in overdoses. Anorexia, blurred vision, headache, hypothermia, vertigo, disorientation, and excessive sedation with lethargy and stupor, hypotension, opisthotonus, tonic-clonic convulsions, coma, respiratory failure and/or vasomotor collapse, frequently sudden, which has been the distinguishing feature in fatal cases of phenothiazine overdosage. Small pupils have been observed more commonly in young children. Late manifestations include bone marrow depresssion, liver damage, and diuresis caused by a toxic effect on the renal tubules.

The ferric chloride test on urine (p. 12) can confirm the diagnosis of phenothiazine overdose, but it may not be positive when only dystonic symptoms are present.

Treatment: Induce emesis (Ipecac Syrup, p. 3) or perform gastric lavage (p. 4). Gastric lavage is indicated up to many hours after ingestion. Unabsorbed phenothiazine is radiopaque in the gastrointestinal tract and may be seen on an x-ray of the abdomen. In patients exhibiting only sedation and extrapyramidal signs, diphenhydramine (Benadryl) 2 mg/kg, intramuscularly or intravenously, is effective. Generally, extrapyramidal signs do not indicate life-threatening toxicity and usually will abate without sequelae, so therapy should be moderate. Patients who ingested large doses and are in a stupor or coma, and/or have hypotension require hospitalization. A balanced hydrating fluid should be used to raise the blood pressure. The patient should be in the head-down position because phenothiazines are alpha-adrenergic blocking agents and cause orthostatic hypotension. Leverternol (Levophed) may be infused if intravenous fluids alone do not raise the arterial blood pressure to normal after the central venous pressure has been restored. Treat convulsions with diazepam (0.05 to 0.1 mg/kg slowly intravenously); phenothiazines potentiate the central nervous system and respiratory depression of barbiturates, sedatives, alcohol, narcotics, and anesthetics. Respiration must be closely monitored. Intubation and artificial ventilation may be required. Exchange transfusion may be lifesaving in infants. Dialysis is not considered beneficial.

References:

Duffy, B.: Acute phenothiazine intoxication in children. Med. J. Aust., 1:676, 1971.

Weisdorf, D., Kramer, J., Goldborg, A., and Klawans, H.L.: Physostigmine for cardiac and neurologic manifestations of phenothiazine poisoning. Clin. Pharmacol. Therap., 24:663, 1978.

Gupta, J.M., and Lovejoy, F.H., Jr.: Acute phenothiazine toxicity in childhood: A five-year survey. Pediatrics, 39:771, 1967.

Niemann, J.T., Stapczynski, J.S., Rothstein, R.J., and Laks, M.M.: Cardiac conduction and rhythm disturbances following suicidal ingestion of mesoridazine. Ann. Emerg. Med., 10:585, 1981.

Solomon, K.: Phenothiazine-induced bulbar palsy-like syndrome and sudden death. Amer. J. Psychiat., 134:308, 1977.

Plants

The growing of plants has become a common hobby in the United States, and plants are the leading substance ingested by children less than 5 years old in reports to the National Clearinghouse for Poison Control Centers since 1977. In this age range, one of every eight ingestions was of a plant.

Table 16 was prepared to provide the physician with a greater awareness of poisonous plants in and about the home. More than 700 known poisonous plants exist in the northern hemisphere, but only the most common ones will be listed here. Nontoxic plants and berries are given on p. 19. Even if plant parts are not toxic, they are a foreign body aspiration and digestive hazard for small children.

Dermatitis is the most common morbidity, with more than one million people contacting dermatitis from plants each year. The most common cause of this type of dermatitis is poison ivy (Rhus Toxicodendron).

The same general principles of treatment apply to a plant ingestion as to any other toxic agent, i.e., removal, dilution, absorption, the use of a few specific antidotes, and general supportive care.

Ipecac Syrup may be used to induce vomiting (p. 3), or a gastric lavage may be performed (p.4). The most common toxic plants, toxic chemicals or substances, symptoms, and specific treatments are given in Table 16.

Reference:

Grote, R.A., Masoud, A.N., and McIntire, M.S.: Plant poisoning in children. Paediatrician, 6:278, 1977.

Table 16
Poisonous Plants

Plants	Scientific Name	Toxic Part or Ingredient	Symptoms and Special Treatment
Houseplants and Cultivated Flowers			
Philodendron Caladium Dumb cane Elephant ear	Philodendron sp. Caladium sp. Dieffenbachia sp. Colocasia sp.	oxalates	Irritation of the buccal mucosa, edema of the pharynx, gastroenteritis; ingestion results in hypocalcemia. **Treatment:** rinse the mouth with milk; calcium salts for hypocalcemia.
Narcissus Amaryllis Daffodil	All are subfamily Amaryllidaseae	the aklaloid lycorine	Vomiting and diarrhea.
Lily-of-the-valley Foxglove Oleander	Convallaria majalis Digitalis purpurea Nerium oleander	cardiac glycosides	Irritation of the mucous membranes, cardiovascular toxicity. **Treatment:** must measure serum potassium and treat if high; further drugs and therapies appropriate to EKG findings.
Monkshood Larkspur	Acontium sp. Delphinium sp.	alkaloid aconitine	Restlessness, salivation, irregular heartbeat. **Treatment:** empty the stomach (see p. 3); atropine for symptoms.
Autumn crocus Glory lily	Colchicum autumnale Gloriosa sp.	colchicine	Gastrointestinal, respiratory, renal, and central nervous system toxicity.
Poinsettia Snow-on-the-mountain	Eupharbia sp.	unknown acrid principle in milky sap	Irritation of mucous membranes and gastrointestinal tract. Poinsetta usually not toxic.
Anemone	Anemone sp.	portoanemonin aglycone	Irritation to mucous membrane, gastroenteritis.

Plants	Scientific Name	Toxic Part or Ingredient	Symptoms and Special Treatment
Iris	Iris sp.	resins like podophyllotoxin	Gastroenteritis.
Jerusalem cherry	Solanum pseudocapsicum	alkaloids	Gastroenteritis, central nervous system depression.

Plants Found as Wild Flowers and Weeds

Plants	Scientific Name	Toxic Part or Ingredient	Symptoms and Special Treatment
Deadly nightshade Black nightshade Climbing nightshade (also called woody or deadly)	Atropa belladonna Solanum nigrum Solanum dulcamara	atropine, solanine, and related glycoalkaloids	Dry mouth; mydriasis and loss of accommodation; hot, flushed skin; hyperthermia: convulsions. **Treatment:** emesis (see p. 3); physostigmine for severe symptoms.
Horse nettle Jimson weed Henbane	Solanum carolinense Datura sp. Hyoscyamus niger	scopolamine	
Green hellebore False hellebore	Veratrum viride Veratrum californicum	venatrum alkaloids	Gastrointestinal irritation; respiratory and cardiovascular depression. **Treatment:** atropine.
Death camus	Zygadenus venenosus		
Pokeweed	Phytolacca sp.	resins like podophyllotoxins	Vomiting, sweating, colic, diarrhea, central nervous system depression.
May apple	Podophyllum sp.	podophylloresin	May produce peripheral neuropathy, vomiting, colic, diarrhea, drowsiness, impaired vision.
Poison ivy Poison oak Poison sumac	Toxicodendron sp.	urshiol	Dermatitis manifested by red, itchy skin and clear blisters that exude serum; if ingested, causes severe mucosal irritation.

Common Name	Scientific Name	Toxic Principle	Symptoms / Treatment
Poison wood			**Treatment:** 1% hydrocortisone lotion or calamine lotion, systemic steroids if severe irritation to mucosa.
Spurges	Euphorbia sp.	unknown acrid principle	Severe irritation to mucosa.
Jack-in-the-pulpit Wild calla Skunk cabbage	Arisaema triphyllum Calla palustris Symplocarpus foetidus	calcium oxalate crystals	Irritation and burning of the mouth. **Treatment:** rinse mouth with milk or magnesium hydroxide.
Water hemlock	Cicuta maculata	cirutoxin	Grand mal seizures. **Treatment:** symptomatic to prevent and control seizures, salivation, vomiting, diarrhea, and convulsions.
Poison hemlock	Conium maculatum	alkaloid coniine	Salivation, nausea, vomiting, diarrhea, sensory disturbance, convulsions, coma; death may occur from respiratory paralysis.
White snakeroot	Eupatorium rugosum	tremetol, may be in milk of a poisoned cow	Weakness, debilitation, vomiting, tremors, and death.
Precatory bean (rosary pea)	Abrus precatorius	phytotoxin abrin	Burning sensation of the mouth and throat, delayed gastroenteritis, depression of vasomotor center, vascular collapse.
Buttercup	Ranuculus sp.	protoanemonin	Gastrointestinal irritation.
Morning glory	Ipomoea violaceae	seeds contain lysergic acid monoethylamide	Central nervous system and psychic stimulation.
Plants Grown in Gardens and As Cultivated Crops			
Potato Tomato	Solanum tuberosum Lycopersicum esculentum	green parts and sprouts contain glycoalkaloids	Gastrointestinal irritation, headache, and central nervous system depression; dermatitis.

Plants	Scientific Name	Toxic Part or Ingredient	Symptoms and Special Treatment
Rhubarb	Rheum rhaponticum	leaves contain oxalate crystals and soluble oxalates	Irritation of oral and gastric mucosa; ingestion results in hypocalcemia with seizures. **Treatment:** rinse mouth with milk; intravenous calcium salts for hypocalcemia.
Tobacco	Nicotiana sp.	nicotine	Salivation; gastroenteritis; large amounts produce convulsions.
Castor bean	Ricinus communis	toxalbumin rican	Burning sensation of the mouth and throat, delayed gastroenteritis, depression of vasomotor center, hepatic injury, hemolysis, convulsions, and death.

Plants Found as Trees and Woody Shrubs

Plants	Scientific Name	Toxic Part or Ingredient	Symptoms and Special Treatment
Cherry trees Apple trees Peach trees Apricot trees Choke cherry trees	Prunus sp. Malus sylvestria Prunus persica Prunus armeniaca Prunus virginiana	leaves and pits or seeds contain glycosides hydrolyzed to hydrocyanic acid	Dyspnea, paralysis, convulsions, coma, and death. **Treatment:** emesis, sodium nitrate intravenously, see p. 149 for cyanide therapy.
Mountain laurel Rhododendrons	Kalmia latifolia Rhododendron sp.	andromedotoxin	Local and gastrointestinal irritation, respiratory and cardiovascular depression. **Treatment:** atropine.
Yew	Taxus sp.	alkaloid taxine	Vomiting, colic, hypotension, respiratory depression.
English holly	Ilex aquifolium	ilexanthin and ilex acid	Vomiting and diarrhea.

Mistletoe	Phoradendron flavescens	berries contain phenethylamines and tyramine	Gastroenteritis and cardiovascular collapse.
Black locust	Robinia pseudoacacia	controversy over toxins, thought to be phyto-toxins and glycosides	Anorexia, weakness, gastroenteritis, dilated pupils, weak and irregular pulse.
Daphne	Daphne sp.	glycoside in which the aglycone is dihydrohycoumarin	Burning and irritation to the skin and gastrointestinal tract, bloody diarrhea, stupor, weakness, and convulsions.

Salicylates
(Aspirin, Sodium Salicylate, Methyl Salicylate)

Type of Product: Analgesic, antipyretic, anti-inflammatory agent.

Ingredients/Description: Aspirin (acetylsalicylic acid) is supplied in tablets of various sizes, most commonly containing 65, 325, 487, 500, or 650 mg. Aspirin is also available as an effervescent tablet or in chewing gum form. Sodium salicylate is supplied as 325 or 625 mg tablets. Both products also come as enteric-coated tablets and are found in cold and analgesic mixtures as tablets, capsules, powder, or liquids.

Methyl salicylate is available as oil of wintergreen (1 ml = 1 gm salicylate equivalent) and as an ingredient in analgesic ointments and liniments.

Homomenthyl salicylate is available as a sunscreen.

Toxicity: The acute toxic dose of sodium salicylate and aspirin is 150 to 200 mg/kg. A dose of more than 500 mg/kg is considered potentially lethal. The mean lethal dose for adults is probably 10 to 30 gm. Serum salicylate levels at various intervals beginning 4 to 6 hours after a single dose of salicylate can be related to expected severity of intoxication.

When ingested, methyl salicylate (oil of wintergreen) is hydrolyzed in the gastrointestinal tract before it is absorbed so the nomogram **does not apply.** Peak levels may be considerably delayed. One milliliter of oil of wintergreen (99% methyl salicylate) is equivalent to a little more than 1 gm of aspirin in salicylate potency.

Phenyl salicylate is hydrolyzed, probably in the tissues, releasing phenol, the symptoms of which predominate in an overdose.

Homomenthyl salicylate is hydrolyzed to menthol and salicylic acid (46%).

Salicylates are metabolized by hepatic pathways that become saturated in overdose situations. Little free drug is ionized in acid urine, so it is reabsorbed. Increasing urine pH from 7.5 to 8.5 allows excretion of 20 times as much salicylate.

The most serious cases of salicylate intoxication in children result from delay in obtaining treatment (over 12 hours), ingestion of oil of wintergreen, or the therapeutic use of excessive doses (for body weight or state of illness), or too frequent doses over a period of days (chronic).

There is little correlation between the serum salicylate level and the severity of illness in chronic poisoning. Salicylate may be sequestered in the central nervous system and cause selective hypoglycemia of brain tissue or cerebral hemorrhage.

Symptoms and Findings: Salicylates are direct respiratory stimulants, uncouple oxidative phosphorylation and inhibit Krebs cycle enzymes, inhibit amino acid metabolism, and interfere with homeostatic mechanisms, thereby causing

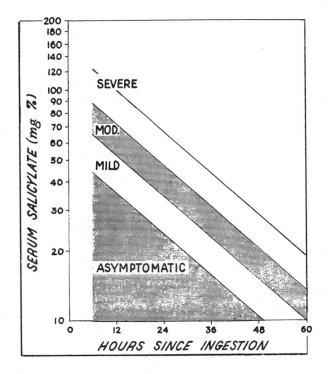

Nomogram relating serum salicylate concentration and expected severity of intoxication at various intervals following the ingestion of a single dose of salicylate. (From Done, A. K.: Salicylate intoxication: Significance of measurements of salicylate in blood in cases of acute ingestion. Pediatrics, 26:800, 1960.

hyperthermia, increased cardiac output, and disturbances in acid-base balance and in plasma electrolytes.

At serum salicylate levels greater than 30 mg/dl, approximately half the patients in single-dose exposures may experience nausea. Vomiting may occur early and be persistent in both acute and chronic intoxication.

As a result of the direct respiratory stimulation, hyperpnea and hyperventilation are prominent, resulting in a carbon dioxide loss and respiratory alkalosis. In adults and older children, the alkalosis may persist until terminal respiratory failure develops. In young children, this phase may rapidly proceed to metabolic acidosis. Associated with this may be serious dehydration and electrolyte imbalance. Transient hyperglycemia and glycosuria are common; however, small children may develop life-threatening hypoglycemia. Some complications that may occur are: hemorrhagic diathesis from inhibition of prothrombin production or thrombocytopenia, oliguria as a result of inappropriate ADH secretion, hyponatremia or inadequate hydration, transient renal failure, or cerebral or pulmonary edema.

Symptoms that may develop after an asymptomatic period include: hyperpnea, vomiting, headache, tinnitus, irritability, restlessness, delirium, hallucinations, confusion, mania, convulsions, coma. Sweating, fever, and dehydration may occur. Death results from respiratory failure, cardiovascular collapse, electrolyte imbalance, or complications.

Treatment: For an ingestion of 100 mg/kg or more, induce emesis (Ipecac Syrup, p. 3) or perform a gastric lavage (p. 4). After evacuation of the stomach, administer activated charcoal (p. 4) and a saline cathartic (p. 5). Significant amounts of salicylate may be present in patients who ingested large overdoses, even 12 hours after ingestion. Obtain blood for salicylate level, pH, pCO_2, bicarbonate, sodium, potassium, chloride, and glucose. Done's nomogram may assist in evaluating the severity of intoxication if the salicylate was ingested in a single dose. Give fluids, electrolytes, and glucose as required to correct dehydration, acidosis, and hypoglycemia. If the patient is in shock, give blood plasma or albumin (10 to 15 ml/kg) immediately. Children less than 4 years old with serious poisoning are usually acidotic on admission to the hospital. Most patients seen within 4 to 6 hours of ingestion of a single dose of 100 to 300 mg of salicylate per kilogram can be treated in the emergency room until repeat serum salicylate levels establish a downward trend and are under 30 mg/dl. Establish good urine flow. Sodium bicarbonate may be given for acidosis either by adding it to the intravenous fluids at a concentration of 15 mEq/l or in individual intravenous doses (3 to 5 mEq/kg) over a 2- to 4-hour period, and repeated cautiously as indicated by response. Monitor blood gases, electrolytes, salicylate levels, and urine pH. In children more than 4 years old, the serum bicarbonate concentration may be low, but the pH of the blood is normal or high (alkalotic). This is caused by stimulation of the respiratory center and a resultant respiratory alkalosis superimposed on a metabolic acidosis. In this situation, bicarbonate must be administered more cautiously. Acetazolamide (Diamox) has been advocated by some to be used in a dose of 5 mg/kg per 24 hours along with bicarbonate therapy. However, it may increase central nervous system salicylate levels. The aim of bicarbonate therapy is to maintain the blood pH within the normal range and the urine pH above 7.5. When urine output is adequate, add KCl to intravenous fluids at a concentration of 30 to 35 mEq/l. The usual fluid requirement during the period of severe symptoms is 2.3 to 4.0 l/M^2 per day. In severe acidosis, large amounts of sodium bicarbonate may be required to correct the acid-base balance. Tetany should be treated by cessation of alkali therapy and intravenous administration of calcium gluconate. Respiratory depression may require artificial ventilation and oxygen. Convulsions may be controlled with diazepam. Reduce hyperpyrexia with external cooling. Vitamin K$_1$ oxide may be given parenterally in doses of 15 mg to prevent hypoprothrombinemia.

The use of dialysis (extracorporal or peritoneal) may be indicated in patients with high salicylate levels (above the "severe" line on the nomogram). Peritoneal dialysis fluid should contain 5% albumin and electrolytes equivalent to normal plasma values. The use of acetazolamide in infants is controversial, and it can make the acidosis more profound.

In the treatment of chronic aspirin poisoning, central nervous system symptoms may resolve more slowly than acid-base derangement. Salicylate levels in spinal fluid may be determined and removal by ion-trapping may be considered (elevate blood pH by continuous drip sodium bicarbonate).

References:

Done, A.K.: Salicylate intoxication. Significance of measurements of salicylate in blood in cases of acute ingestion. Pediatrics, 26:800, 1960.

Brem, J., Pereli, E.M., Gopalan, S.K., and Miller, T.B.: Salicylism, hyperventilation, and the central nervous system. J. Pediat., 83:264, 1973.

Hill, J.B.: Salicylate intoxication. New Engl. J. Med., 288:1110, 1973.

Buchanan, N., Kundig, H., and Eyberg, C.: Experimental salicylate intoxication in young baboons. J. Pediat., 86:225, 1975.

Thurston, J.H., Pollock, P.G., Warren, S.K., and Jones, E.M.: Reduced brain glucose with normal plasma glucose in salicylate poisoning. J. Clin. Invest., 49:2139, 1970.

Temple, A.R.: Acute and chronic effects of aspirin toxicity and their treatment. Arch. Intern. Med., 141:364, 1981.

Theophylline

Type of Product: Antiasthmatic drug.

Ingredients/Description: Available as liquid, tablet, capsule, and intravenous solution (as aminophylline). Concentrations of oral liquid range from 5 to 20 mg/ml. Tablets range from 100 to 300 mg, and capsules range from 60 to 250 mg. Sustained-release capsules and tablets are available. The intravenous solution contains 25 mg/ml.

There are a variety of theophylline derivatives yielding varying percentages of anhydrous theophylline. The most common is aminophylline (theophylline ethylenediamine), which is converted to approximately 85% by weight anhydrous theophylline. Others with their conversions to theophylline are:

anhydrous theophylline	approximately 100%
aminophylline hydrous	approximately 80%
choline theophylline	approximately 64%
theophylline calcium salicylate	approximately 50%
theophylline monohydrate	approximately 91%
theophylline olamine	approximately 75%
theophylline sodium acetate	approximately 60%
theophylline sodium glycinate	approximately 46%

Elixophyllin is a preparation containing free theophylline

dissolved in 20% ethanol. Diphylline is a derivative which is not converted to theophylline and is excreted unchanged in the urine. Theo-Dur Sprinkle contains anhydrous theophylline microencapsulated in a polymer. It comes in 50, 75, 125, and 200 mg oversized capsules which are meant to be opened.

Toxicity: Acute doses of theophylline greater than 10 mg/kg may produce mild toxicity, and doses greater than 20 mg/kg may be expected to cause symptoms. Toxicity is generally serum-concentration related: therapeutic, 10 to 20 μg/ml; mild toxicity, 20 to 40 μg/ml; severe toxicity, 40 to 80 μg/ml.

Serum levels can be estimated from a single exposure by doubling the milligram per kilogram theophylline dose. The elimination rate of theophylline varies considerably among individuals and in the presence of some drugs. It is eliminated from the body primarily through hepatic metabolism. Only about 7% of free theophylline is excreted by the kidney.

Symptoms and Findings: Mild toxicity includes nausea, vomiting, headache, irritability, insomnia, and tremulousness. Abdominal cramps and diarrhea have been noted. Severe toxicity includes protracted vomiting with hematemesis, restlessness, agitation, and convulsions. Arrhythmias may occur.

Treatment: Induce emesis (Ipecac Syrup, p. 3) or perform a gastric lavage (p. 4) followed by activated charcoal (p. 4) and a saline laxative (p. 5). Obtain a plasma theophylline level and monitor until levels reach the therapeutic range. Treat mild toxicity expectantly with reassurance and mild sedation. Repeated dosing of activated charcoal has been shown to reduce the serum half-life and increase total body clearance of theophylline. Provide full supportive care, including cardiac monitoring and adequate hydration with replacement of potassium.

Although seizures may be controlled with diazepam (0.1 to 0.3 mg/kg, intravenously), animal studies suggest that phenobarbital has the advantage of stimulating the enzymatic metabolism of the theophylline.

When blood theophylline levels are greater than 60 μg/ml, or if severe or prolonged toxicity is evident, peritoneal dialysis, hemodialysis, or charcoal hemoperfusion should be considered. Phenytoin and carbamazepine in individual cases have markedly reduced half-life and increased clearance of theophylline.

References:

Zwillich, C.W., Sutton, F.D., Jr., Neff, T.A., *et al.:* Theophylline induced seizures in adults: Correlation with serum concentrations. Ann. Intern. Med., **82**:784, 1975.

Russo, M.E.: Management of theophylline intoxication with charcoal-column hemoperfusion. New Engl. J. Med., **300**:24, 1979.

Levy, G., Gibson, T.P., Whitman, W., and Procknal, J.: Hemodialysis clearance of theophylline. J.A.M.A., **237**:1466, 1977.

Miceli, J.N., Clay, B., Fleischmann, L.E., Sarnaik, A.P., Aronow, R., and Done, A.K.: Pharmacokinetics of severe theophylline intoxication managed by peritoneal dialysis. Develop. Pharmacol. Therap., **1**:16, 1980.

Berlinger, W.G., Spector, R., Goldberg, M.J., Johnson, G.F., Quee, C.K., and Berg, M.J.: Enhancement of theophylline clearance by oral activated charcoal. Clin. Pharmacol. Therap., **33**:351, 1983.

Marquis, J.F., Carruthers, S.G., Spence, J.D., Brownstone, Y.S., and Toogood, J.H.: Phenytoin-theophylline interaction. New Engl. J. Med., **307**:1189, 1982.

Rosenberry, K.R., Defusco, C.J., Mansmann, H.C., and McGeady, S.J.: Reduced theophylline half-life induced by carbamazepine therapy. J. Pediat., **102**:472, 1983.

Thyroid Hormones

Type of Product: Hormone for replacement therapy.

Ingredients/Description: See Table 17. Check the *Physicians' Desk Reference* for less common preparations.

Toxicity: Thyroid hormones rarely cause toxicity.

Symptoms: A 15-month-old child developed serious poisoning after the ingestion of 3.2 gm (50 tablets) of dessicated thyroid.
Liothyronine (T_3) is better absorbed and has a more rapid onset of action. Massive overdose may result in symptoms within 1 to 4 hours. Ingestion of preparations containing L-thyroxine, including dessicated thyroid, may result in

Table 17
Thyroid Ingredients

Ingredients	Description	Doses Equivalent to 1 Grain Dessicated Thyroid	Trade Name	Tab/Cap Size
Thyroid USP	T_4 and T_3 from dessicated gland	65 mg (1 gr)	various	Cap: 1, 2, 3, 5 gr Tab: 1/4 to 5 gr
Thyroglobulin	T_4 and T_3 from purified thyroid gland	65 mg	Proloid	Tab: 16, 32, 65, 100, 130, 200, 325 mg
Levothyroxin	Synthetic T_4	100 μg	Synthroid	Tab: 25, 50, 100, 150, 200, 300 μg
			Levothroid	Tab: 25, 50, 100, 150, 175, 200, 300, 400, 500 μg
Liothyronine	Synthetic T_3	25 μg	Cytomel	Tab: 5, 25, 50 μg
Liotrix	Synthetic T_4 and T_3 in 4:1 ratio	$T_4/T_3 = 50/12.5$ μg	Thyrolar	Tab: equivalent to 1/4, 1/2, 1, 2, 3 gr dessicated thyroid
		$T_4/T_3 = 60/15$ μg	Euthroid	Tab: equivalent to 1/2, 1, 2, 3 gr dessicated thyroid

symptoms with onset as late as the fifth day. Symptoms may persist for 1 to 2 weeks.

Symptoms include nervousness, irritability, midriasis, diarrhea, flushing, sweating, hyperpyrexia, and depressed reflexes. Cardiac symptoms include palpitation, tachycardia, atrial fibrillation, and ventricular tachycardia; and extrasystoles may be observed.

Moderately elevated doses over a prolonged time may result in symptoms of hyperthyroidism. This usually comes from excessive doses being prescribed, patient-directed weight reduction attempts, or suicide attempts.

Treatment: If a child ingests more than 1,000 μg per M^2 of L-thyroxine or its equivalent, induce emesis (Ipecac Syrup, p. 3) or perform a gastric lavage (p. 4). Administer activated charcoal (p. 4) and a cathartic (p. 5). L-thyroxine (T_4) has an enterohepatic circulation, and repeated doses of activated charcoal may be useful in severely symptomatic patients.

Admit all children who have ingested synthetic hormones in a dose greater than 1,000 μg per M^2 of L-thyroxine; they should be placed on frequent vital sign observation or on a cardiac monitor. If tachycardia of a mild degree occurs, watchful waiting is appropriate. If a faster heart rate or extrasystoles occur, the heart rate should be controlled with propranolol, 1 mg/kg per 24 hours, orally in four doses for children, or 20 to 80 mg four times a day in adults.

Laboratory tests of thyroid function are useful to rule out toxicity if they are normal 4 to 6 hours after ingestion. T_4 levels several times normal may not be associated with symptoms, and patients may be asymptomatic with moderate elevations of T_3 by RIA.

References:

Levy, R.P., and Gilger, W.G.: Acute thyroid poisoning: Report of a case. New Engl. J. Med., 256:459, 1957.

Funderburk, S.J., and Spaulding, J.S.: Sodium levothyroxine (Synthroid R) intoxication in a child. Pediatrics, 45:298, 1970.

Von Hofe, S.E., and Young, R.L.: Thyrotoxicosis after a single ingestion of levothyroxine. J.A.M.A., 237:1361, 1977.

Valente, W.A., Goldiner, W.H., Hamilton, B.P., Wiswell, J.G., and Mersey, J.H.: Thyroid hormone levels after acute L-thyroxine loading in hypothyroidism. J. Clin. Endocrinol. Metab., 53:527, 1981.

Toluene
(Toluol, Methylbenzene, Methylbenzol, Phenylmethane)

Type of Product: Solvent, paint remover, degreaser, pesticide, fuel, urine preservative, and plastic and rubber cements.

Ingredients/Description: A product of the distillation of coal tar. A colorless, highly flammable liquid which burns with a smokey flame. Toluene is an aromatic hydrocarbon.

Toxicity: Toluene is readily absorbed by inhalation and ingestion. It has a greater acute toxicity than benzene. Aspiration of small amounts may be fatal. Exposure to vapors at 600 to 800 ppm for 3 to 8 hours has produced central nervous system stimulation followed by depression similar to alcohol intoxication. Toluene is rapidly metabolized to benzoic acid, which then is conjugated with glycine in the liver and excreted in the urine as hippuric acid. Methods are available to determine blood and breath toluene concentrations.

Symptoms and Findings: Toluene is an irritant to mucous membranes, skin, and eyes. Ingestion is likely to cause a burning sensation in the mouth and stomach, nausea, salivation, vomiting, substernal pain, cough, and hoarseness. Dermal exposure can cause a burning sensation, local irritation, and possibly blistering of the skin. Eye exposures possibly can cause burns. Inhalation may result in bronchial and laryngeal irritation, transient euphoria, headache, giddiness, vertigo, ataxia, and renal tubular acidosis. At higher doses, narcosis, confusion, and coma may occur, with hematuria, proteinuria, and eosinophilia. Continued contact can cause respiratory failure or cardiac arrhythmias. Chronic exposure to toluene may cause hepatic, encephalopathic, and renal toxicity.

Treatment: With inhalation, remove the patient from the source of exposure, stabilize or establish respirations, and reassure the patient. Inhalation of toluene can result in metabolic acidosis with a high anion gap that can be treated with sodium bicarbonate and/or potassium chloride to restore

:trolyte balance. Epinephrine may induce life-threatening hythmias.

Decontaminate the skin if needed (p. 6). If the product gets into the eyes, injury may be transient if decontamination is carried out immediately (p. 6).

If toluene is ingested, emesis should be initiated with Ipecac Syrup unless this procedure is contraindicated (p. 3); in which case, perform a gastric lavage (p. 4); follow with activated charcoal (p. 4). Institute supportive care. Do not use epinephrine (p. 145). Treat symptomatically.

References:

Gosselin, R.E., Hodge, H.C., Smith, R.P., and Gleason, M.N.: Clinical Toxicology of Commercial Products, ed. 4. Baltimore: Williams and Wilkins, Sect. III, pp. 320-323, 1976, reprinted 1977.

Knox, J.W., and Nelson, J.R.: Permanent encephalopathy from toluene inhalation. New Engl. J. Med., 275:1494, 1966.

Taher, S.M., Anderson, R.J., McCartney, R., Popovtzer, M.M., and Schrier, R.W.: Renal tubular acidosis associated with toluene "sniffing." New Engl. J. Med., 290:765, 1974.

Streicher, H.Z., Gabow, P.A., Moss, A.H., Kono, D., and Kaehny, W.D.: Syndromes of toluene sniffing in adults. Ann. Intern. Med., 94:758, 1981.

Garriott, J.C., Foerster, E., Juarez, L., De La Garza, F., Mendiola, I., and Curoe, J.: Measurement of toluene in blood and breath in cases of solvent abuse. Clin. Toxicol., 18:471, 1981.

Tricyclic Antidepressants

Type of Product: Antidepressant.

Ingredients/Description: Many different antidepressant products are available. Some contain only tricyclic antidepressants (e.g., Elavil, Sinequan); others are combination products (e.g., Etrafon, Triavil). Tablets may contain 10, 25, 50, 75, 100, or 150 mg of the tricyclic. The variety of tricyclic compounds include: (1) Tertiary amines: amitriptyline (Amitid, Amitril, Elavil, Endep, SK-Pramine, Tofranil, Antipress, Imavate, Presamine); doxepin (Adapin, Sinequan); trimipramine (Surmontil). (2) Secondary amines: amoxapine (Asendin); nortriptyline (Aventyl HCl, Pamelor); desipramine (Norpramin, Petrofane); protriptyline (Vivactil).

Toxicity: Toxic effects are not necessarily dose dependent. Toxic effects have been noted after ingestion of one tablet in a child. Observation of clinical effects should determine the course of treatment regardless of the dose. A QRS duration of 100 msec or greater within the first 24 hours following the overdose is an indication of a major overdose. Anticholinergic or central nervous system effects may not be evident before the onset of serious cardiac arrhythmias. In contrast, large overdoses of amoxapine have resulted in severe seizure activity, metabolic acidosis, and coma without the cardiac complications.

Symptoms and Findings: Tricyclic antidepressants are rapidly distributed once they are absorbed. They are highly lipophilic, become protein bound, and have a tremendously large volume of distribution of 15 to 40 l/kg. Toxicity is generally caused by an atropine-like anticholinergic effect, blockade of reuptake of norepinephrine, and a direct myocardial depressant effect. A patient with a history of a tricyclic antidepressant overdose may have a clinical presentation varying from minor anticholinergic signs and symptoms and lethargy to severe symptomatology with coma, seizures, lethal ventricular dysrhythmias, respiratory depression, and cardiac arrest. Overdoses are also associated with hypertension, hypotension, shock, abnormal deep tendon reflexes, hypothermia, hyperthermia, choreoathetosis, myoclonus, and death.

Treatment: Even hours after the ingestion, the stomach should be emptied. Induce emesis (Ipecac Syrup, p. 3) unless contraindicated; in which case, perform a gastric lavage (p. 4). After lavage or emesis, activated charcoal and a saline laxative should be instilled via the lavage tube or given by mouth (p. 4, 5). The administration of activated charcoal is recommended every 4 to 6 hours for 24 to 48 hours, depending on the overdose, to prevent recycling of the drug in the body. Patients with a tricyclic poisoning but few signs and symptoms on arrival should be observed for increasing toxicity from the delayed gastrointestinal absorption of the drug. They should be observed for development of cardiotoxicity, respiratory depression and/or central nervous system toxicity before being discharged. QRS complexes equal to or greater than 100 msec correlate with tricyclic (including active metabolites) plasma levels of 1,000 ng/ml or greater and indicate a medically serious overdose. (Lower levels of amoxapine may be significant.) No correlation has been found between neurologic symptoms and the development of cardiotoxic symptoms. Cardiac monitoring is necessary and should be continued until the patient is dysrhythmia free for at least 24 hours.

There is not uniformity of medical opinion about specific treatment, but it appears that the use of sodium bicarbonate intravenously to bring the blood pH up to 7.5 has an important primary role in potentially serious tricyclic overdose except for amoxapine. The salutory effects relate to decreased myocardial sensitivity to arrhythmias, an ability to maintain or drive potassium back into myocardial cells, increased binding of the drug to plasma proteins (making it biologically inactive), and correction of respiratory or metabolic acidosis. The disadvantage would be in imipramine overdose, where theoretically there may be an increased central nervous system uptake of the drug in the presence of elevated blood pH.

Physostigmine (adult: 1 to 2 mg intravenously slowly over 2 minutes; child: 0.5 mg intravenously slowly over 2 minutes; may repeat every 20 to 30 minutes for either child or adult) may be used early in the course cautiously to reverse anticholinergic symptoms, as a confirmatory diagnostic aid or to treat hypotension, hypertension, cardiac arrhythmias, and delirium not responsive to alkalization and volume expansion.

Of the antidysrhythmic drugs available, phenytoin appears to be indicated for treatment of first degree A-V block and/or intraventricular conduction delay. A dose of 5 to 7 mg/kg given intravenously, not to exceed 50 mg per minute or a total of 500 mg in adults, has been recommended. Other medications possibly indicated are lidocaine, norepinephrine, and, for seizure control, diazepam.

Electrolytes should be monitored, and potassium replaced cautiously.

Dialysis and diuresis appear to offer little benefit.

References:

Biggs, J.T., Spiker, D.G, Petit, J.M., and Ziegler, V.E.: Tricyclic antidepressant overdose: Incidence of symptoms. J.A.M.A., **238**:135, 1977.

Robinson, D., and Barker, M.: Tricyclic antidepressant cardiotoxicity. J.A.M.A., **236**:2089, 1976.

Rumack, B.H.: Anticholinergic poisoning. Treatment with physostig-
mine. Pediatrics, **52**:449, 1973.
Hagerman, G.A., and Hanashiro, P.K.: Reversal of tricyclic-antidepres-
sant-induced cardiac conduction abnormalities by phenytoin. Ann.
Emerg. Med., **10**:82, 1981.
Pentel, P., and Sioris, L.: Incidence of late arrhythmias following
tricyclic antidepressant overdose. Clin. Toxicol., **18**:543, 1981.
Hoffman, J.R., and McElroy, C.R.: Bicarbonate therapy for dys-
rhythmia and hypotension in tricyclic antidepressant overdose.
Western J. Med., **134**:60, 1981.
Browne, J.L., Tsuang, M.T., and Perry, P.J.: Amoxapine neurotoxicity:
A case report with long-term following. Drug Intell. Clin. Pharm.,
16:404, 1982.

Warfarin

Type of Product: Anticoagulant, rodenticide.

Ingredients/Description: d-Con Rat and Mouse Poison contains
warfarin, 0.025%. Other rodenticides contain warfarin in concentrations as high as 0.5%. Talon Rodenticide contains bro-
difacoum (40 times more potent than warfarin) as the active
ingredient.

Toxicity: Warfarin induces bleeding by inhibiting prothrombin
formation. Bleeding secondary to inhibition of prothrombin
results only after prothrombin supplies are depleted. Thus,
multiple doses generally are required before bleeding diathesis occurs. It causes no problem in children on a single,
acute ingestion unless enormous amounts are consumed.

Symptoms and Findings: Onset of bleeding is usually 24 to 36
hours after the first of several doses. Prolongation of the
prothrombin time is the main manifestation leading clinically to hematemesis, epistaxis, bleeding from the skin,
mucous membranes, gastrointestinal tract, and genitourinary tract (blood in urine and feces).

Treatment: The average child eating a few mouthfuls of 0.025
to 0.05% rat bait at a single sitting is generally not at risk,
and no treatment is required.

  If the ingestion is large or repeated doses have been
consumed, vitamin K_1 should be given (1 to 5 mg intra-

muscularly for a child, and 10 mg intramuscularly for an adult) and may need to be repeated. If toxicity as manifest by bleeding occurs, restoration of the prolonged prothrombin level to normal should be considered with the use of exchange transfusion. Do not induce vomiting, perform gastric lavage, or give cathartics because these procedures may induce internal bleeding or hemorrhage. Further absorption can be prevented by giving activated charcoal.

References:

Dreisbach, R.H.: Handbook of Poisoning, ed. 10. Los Altos, California: Lange Medical Publishers, 1980.

Gosselin, R.E., Hodge, H.C., Smith, R.P., and Gleason, M.N.: Clinical Toxicology of Commercial Products, ed. 4. Baltimore: Williams and Wilkins, Sect. III, pp. 317-320, 1976, reprinted 1977.

Shearer, M.J., and Barkhan, P.: Vitamin K_1 and therapy of massive warfarin overdose. Lancet, 1:266, 1979.

Formulary for the Emergency Room or Clinic Treatment of Poisoned Patients

Drugs	How Supplied		Poison	Indications and Tactics of Administration	Contraindications (C) and Adverse Reactions (A)
	Dose Form	Amount and Concentration			
Amyl nitrate	Pearles (replace yearly)	0.18 ml	Cyanide Hydrogen sulfide	Give one pearle as inhalant for 30 seconds of each 2 minutes while preparing NaNO$_2$ and sodium thiosulfate IV solutions	C-Do not use sodium thiosulfate for H$_2$S.
Antivenin, Black widow, (latrodectus antivenom)	Vial	2.5 ml	Black widow spider, Northern widow spider	Skin test before administration; 1 vial deeply IM, rare second dose required.	C-Usually only needed for the very young or older patient. A-Various allergic responses to horse serum; treat with epinephrine or diphenhydramine.
Antivenin (Crotalidae)	Vial	10 ml	Rattlesnake, copperhead, cottonmouth	Skin or conjunctival test before 3-5 10 ml vials diluted in 100 to 500 ml of IV fluid given IV drip over 1 hour; 3-20 vials may be necessary over the next 6 hours; monitor circumference of extremity 10 cm proximal to bite and at another proximal site every 15-30 minutes as a guide to antivenin administration.	C-Never inject antivenin into finger or toe. A-Various allergic responses to horse serum; treat with epinephrine or diphenhydramine.

Drugs	How Supplied		Poison	Indications and Tactics of Administration	Contraindications (C) and Adverse Reactions (A)
	Dose Form	Amount and Concentration			
Atropine sulfate	Ampule	1 ml (0.3 mg/ml) (0.4 mg/ml) (0.5 mg/ml)	Cholinesterase inhibitors (organophosphate and carbamate pesticides), physostigmine, pilocarpine	Overcome cyanosis first, then the usual starting IV dose is 0.5 mg for a child and 2 mg for an older child or adult. Repeat every 3 to 10 minutes as needed. Requires titration until atropinization is achieved as indicated by the cessation of secretions and/or heart rate >180 per minute. Large total doses may be required in organophosphate poisoning. For physostigmine and pilocarpine toxicity, an initial dose of 0.01 mg/kg should be used.	C–Cyanosis. A–Mucous membrane dryness; dilated pupils, rapid pulse and respiration, restlessness, irritability, disorientation, hallucination, medullary depression, elevated temperature.
	Vial	20 ml (0.4 mg/ml) 30 ml (0.5 mg/ml)			
Calcium gluconate 10%	Ampule	10 ml (1 gm)	Fluoride, chlorinated hydrocarbons, oxalates, detergents, widow spider bites	For hypocalcemic tetany, inject very slowly IV. Adult: 10-20 ml per dose. Child: 1-2 ml per dose. Monitor for cardiac arrhythmias.	A–Cardiac arrest.
			Hydrofluoric acid	Infiltrate area of exposure (if hand, advise only being done by someone familiar with the anatomy of the hand)	

Charcoal, activated	Powder	pound or kilogram boxes	General adsorbent; little effect with metals, alcohols, boric acid, corrosives, cyanide, and hydrocarbons	If Ipecac Syrup is used, give after emesis. Completely nontoxic, so err on large side of dose. Give at least 10 gm to children and 30 gm to adults. May be repeated. Slurry with water. Do not slurry with milk, ice cream, or other food which will bind to it. Give by cup, straw, or nasogastric tube.	A-Difficult to remove from clothing.
Chlorpromazine (Thorazine)	Ampule	1 ml or 2 ml (25 mg/ml)	Amphetamine	Sedate patient with a 0.5-1 mg/kg IM (for amphetamine and barbiturate combined overdose, use ½ dose of chlorpromazine). May control convulsions or be used to prevent severe hyperexcitability and agitation caused by amphetamines. Do not use for treatment of toxicity associated with chronic amphetamine abuse.	A-May have additive affect with central nervous system depressants. A-May cause orthostatic hypotension. C-Do not use in comatose patients with cardiovascular or liver disease. C-Do not use when STP, MDA, or other than USP amphetamines have been or are suspected to have been ingested.
Deferoxamine mesylate (Desferal)	Vial	(500 gm)	Iron overdose	IM: add 2 ml water for injection, then draw up dose and administer. IV: add dose to 0.9% saline, 5% glucose in water or Ringer's lactate for IV rate not to exceed 15 mg/kg per hour. Initial dose:	C-Severe renal disease or anuria. A-Too rapid administration may cause hypotension and shock; may have flushing and urticaria.

Drugs	How Supplied		Poison	Indications and Tactics of Administration	Contraindications (C) and Adverse Reactions (A)
	Dose Form	Amount and Concentration			
				0.5-1.0 gm; repeat as needed every 4-6 hours, not to exceed the rate of 15 mg/kg per hour or 6 gm total per 24 hours.	
Diazepam (Valium)	Ampule	2 ml (5 mg/ml)	For seizure control	For convulsions and excitement. Adults: 5-10 mg IV, depending on response; may be repeated in 1-4 hours. Children: 0.1-0.3 mg/kg IV, slowly.	A-Hypotension, respiratory arrest or depression, dizziness, vertigo, ataxia, increased cough reflex, laryngospasm, neutropenia, jaundice, urinary retention.
Dimercaprol (BAL)	Ampule	3 ml, 10% solution in oil (100 mg/ml)	Arsenic, lead, mercury, antimony, gold, bismuth, nickel poisoning	3-4 mg/kg per dose IM every 4 hours for 3-7 days as needed.	C-Do not administer iron supplements concurrently; BAL-Fe complex toxic. Use caution if hepatic dysfunction or renal insufficiency are present. A-May cause hemolysis in total G_6PD-deficient patients; tachycardia, elevated blood pressure, nausea, vomiting, abdominal pain, headache, burning in lips, mouth, throat, penis, tingling of hands, sweating.

Diphenhydramine (Benadryl)	Vial Ampule	10 ml and 30 ml (10 mg/ml) 1 ml (50 mg/ml)	Butyrophenones, phenothiazines (idiosyncratic response only)	Adult: 2.5 to 5 mg/kg per dose, IV slowly or IM, not to exceed 100 mg. Child: 2 mg/kg IV slowly or IM, not to exceed 50 mg; 5 mg/kg per 24 hours, IV slowly or IM divided into four doses, not to exceed 300 mg in 24 hours.	A-Drowsiness, hemolytic anemia, anaphylactic reaction.
Dopamine (Intropin)	Ampule	5 ml (40 mg/ml)	For cardiogenic hypotension	For shock, dilute ampule in 250 or 500 ml D$_5$W or 0.9% saline IV drip starting at 2.5 μg/kg per minute, up to 10-20 μg/kg per minute if necessary. The higher infusion rate should not be maintained for longer than 1 hour. Monitor urine flow.	A-Nausea, vomiting, tachycardia, ectopic beats, precordial pain, dyspnea, headache, hypertension, azotemia. C-Tachyarrhythmias, pheochromocytoma, patients taking monoamine oxidase inhibitors.
Epinephrine	1 ml ampule	aqueous solution 1:1,000	Anaphylactic reactions secondary to insect stings or other causes	SC or IV administration. 1 yr: 0.01 ml/kg (maximum, 0.1 ml). 2 yr: 0.1 ml. 5 yr: 0.3 ml. 10 yr: 0.3-0.5 ml. 15 yr: 0.5 ml. Adult: 0.5-1.0 ml. May repeat in 15 min.	A-Tachycardia and palpitation, fear, anxiety, tenseness, restlessness, headache, tremor, weakness, dizziness, pallor, respiratory difficulty, cerebral hemorrhage, cardiac arrhythmias.

Note: Some examples of poisonings in which epinephrine is contraindicated because life-threatening arrhythmias may be induced:
tricyclic antidepressants
some antihistamines
chlorinated hydrocarbons
carbon tetrachloride
2, 4-D

(cont. on p. 146)

| Drugs | How Supplied | | Poison | Indications and Tactics of Administration | Contraindications (C) and Adverse Reactions (A) |
	Dose Form	Amount and Concentration			
		(see p. 145)	diphenhydramine tripelenamine d-chlorpheniramine mercurial diuretics digitalis preparations nitrogen oxides reserpine thyroid hormones organophosphates	heptachlor lindane chlordane toxaphane kerosene xylene chlorpromazine carbamates	
Ethanol	Vial	95% 50%	Methanol or ethylene glycol	Dose to saturate alcohol dehydrogenase in liver, maintain blood alcohol level 100-150 mg% (mg/dl). Loading dose: 1-1.6 ml/kg per OS 50% solution. IV: 7.6 ml/kg 10% ETOH over 30-60 minutes	C-Give glucose first to overcome or prevent hypoglycemia. A-Inebriation, respiratory depression, hypoglycemia (monitor blood glucose levels).
	IV solution Spirits, ferment	10% 80 proof = 40%		Maintenance dose: Start concurrent with loading dose (monitor blood ETOH levels). Oral: 0.3 ml/kg per hour 50% ETOH or IV: 1.4 ml/kg per hour 10% ETOH in D₅W as a drip. Duration to maintain depends on agent and circumstances.	

Drug	Supply		Indication	Dose	Remarks
Ipecac Syrup	Bottle	15 and 30 ml	Whenever an emetic is indicated	Oral dose: 1-5 yr: 15 ml (½ oz, 1 tbsp). >5 yr: 30 ml (1 oz, 2 tbsp). Give followed by 1-2 glassfuls (15 ml/kg) of water to an alert patient with intact gag reflex. Expect emesis in 15-20 minutes; if it does not occur, repeat dose once. Double dose is not toxic.	C-Do not give to comatose or convulsing patient; or following caustic ingestion. Pregnancy is not a contra-indication. A-May not be effective if symptomatic after phenothiazine, antihistamine, or other antiemetic ingestion. Causes drowsiness of mild nature. May lead to repeated vomiting over a 2-3 hour period. Serious side effects of Ipecac Syrup are rare.
Magnesium sulfate (Sodium sulfate)	Ampule 50% solution Epsom Salt	2 ml and 10 ml (500 mg/ml) (1 gm/2 ml) (3 gm/tsp)	1. orally ingested toxicant for which cathartic is indicated 2. Barium compounds, rodenticides, depilatories, fireworks	Oral dose—250 mg/kg (crystals) Oral Doses—(50% solution) 1 yr: 2 gm in 4 ml 2 yr: 2.5 gm in 5 ml 5 yr: 3.7 gm in 7.5 ml 10 yr: 5 gm in 10 ml Adult: 10-30 gm in 20-60 ml If no defecation in 4-5 hours, use suppository to start action 2a. orally to precipitate in stomach 2b. emesis or lavage 2c. 10% Na_2SO_4, 10 ml slowly IV Repeat every 15 min until symptoms subside	C-Renal failure.

Drugs	How Supplied		Poison	Indications and Tactics of Administration	Contraindications (C) and Adverse Reactions (A)
	Dose Form	Amount and Concentration			
Methylene blue	Ampule	10 ml of 1% M.B. solution (10 mg/ml)	Nitrate or nitrite overdose, methemoglobinemia	Give 1-2 ml/10 kg body weight IV slowly over 5-10 min. Repeat dose in 1 hour if needed.	C-Cyanide poisoning. A-Avoid perivenous infiltration, which may cause tissue necrosis; may cause hemolysis in G_6PD-deficient patient.
N-acetyl-cysteine (Mucomyst)	Vial	20% 4, 10, or 30 ml	Acetaminophen	Dilute 4:1 with acidic juice, cola drink, or water just prior to administering orally. Loading dose: 140 mg/kg; then 4 hours later start: Maintenance dose: 70 mg/kg every 4 hours for 17 doses.	C-More than 24 hours post-ingestion or in the presence of liver failure. A-Nausea, vomiting, loose stools.
Naloxone (Narcan)	Ampule	1 ml (0.4 mg/ml), do not use Narcan Neonatal	Narcotic O.D., mixed drug O.D.	Give usual adult dose of 0.4-0.8 mg (1-4 ampules) IV (or 0.01 mg/kg IV). May be given IM or SC if no IV site available. Readminister every 20-60 minutes as necessary to prevent respiratory depression. In overdose of codeine, propoxyphene or pentazocine, larger doses are necessary. Give 2-4 mg (5-10 ampules) IV push (child, use initial dose of 0.01 mg/kg IV; if no response, give 0.1 mg/kg).	Admit pediatric patients to ICU. C-Use with caution in patients with arrhythmias. C-Administer cautiously to patients (and newborn infants of suspect mothers) who may be opiod dependent, to avoid acute withdrawal anginal pain. C-Long-standing bronchial asthma and significant emphysema, shock, hyperthyroidism, hypertension.

Drug	Form	Size	Indication	Dosage	Comments
Physostigmine salicylate (Antilirium)	Ampule	2 ml (1 mg/ml)	1. Antihistamines Belladonna atropine hyoscyamine hyoscyamus scopolamine stramonium 2. Tricyclic antidepressants	Adults: slowly IV 2 mg, repeat 1-4 mg when needed at 20- to 60-minute intervals. Children: 0.5 mg IV, repeat when needed at 20-minute intervals (have atropine ready at ½ the physostigmine dose to reverse physostigmine cholinergic crises).	C-Bradycardia asthmatic attack: urinary tract obstruction, mechanical obstruction of gastrointestinal tract call for caution in use. A-Nausea, vomiting, epigastric pain, miosis, salivation, sweating, lacrimation, dyspnea, bronchospasm, central nervous system stimulant, restlessness, irregular pulse, palpitations, hallucinations, muscular twitching, convulsions.
Pralidoxime (Protopam, 2-PAM)	Vial	1 gm with 20 ml diluent	Organophosphate cholinesterase inhibitors	Adults: 1-2 gm; children: 25-50 mg/kg. IV over 5-10 minutes; repeat at 12 hours if needed. For use in serious poisoning only; always follows atropine. Should be given within 12 hours following exposure.	C-Myasthenia gravis; carbamate poisoning; patients receiving morphine, theophylline, aminophylline, succinylcholine, reserpines, phenothiazines. A-Dizziness, blurred vision, diplopia, tachycardia, headache.
Pyridoxine hydrochloride (Hexa-Betalin)	Vial	10 ml (100 mg/ml)	Isoniazid	1 gm for each gram INH or, if unknown, 5 gm as IV bolus slowly over 5 min. May repeat in 5-10 min.	C-Sensitivity to pyridoxine or ingredients in preparation.
Sodium nitrite (NaNO₂)	Ampule (Lilly Cyanide Antidote Kit)	(300 mg/10 ml)	Cyanide, hydrogen sulfide	Give 1 ampule (300 mg) IV over 3-4 minutes as soon as possible. Speed is essential. If symptoms recur in ½ hour, repeat dose (see pediatric dose on p. 150)	C-Do not use in conjunction with methylene blue. A-If hypotension occurs, epinephrine may be used.

Drugs	How Supplied		Poison	Indications and Tactics of Administration	Contraindications (C) and Adverse Reactions (A)
	Dose Form	Amount and Concentration			
Sodium thiosulfate	Ampule (Lilly Cyanide Antidote Kit)	(12.5 gm/50 ml)	Cyanide	Inject 50 ml IV **after** NaNO$_2$ administration.	C-Hydrogen sulfide poisoning.

Note—**Pediatric Dosage for Cyanide**: Exceeding These May Cause Fatal Methemoglobinemia

Hemoglobin concentration (gm)	Initial Dose 3% NaNO$_2$ (ml/kg IV)	Initial Dose 25% Sodium Thiosulfate (ml/kg IV)
8	0.22 (6.6 mg/kg)	1.10
10	0.27 (8.3 mg/kg)	1.35
12	0.33 (10.0 mg/kg)	1.65
14	0.39 (11.6 mg/kg)	1.95

Drugs	How Supplied		Poison	Indications and Tactics of Administration	Contraindications (C) and Adverse Reactions (A)
Tincture of Green Soap	If not available, mix liquid hand soap and ethanol or isopropanol, 2:1	—	Greasy or oily poisons on the skin; particularly useful with insecticide contamination	Toxin on skin: wash all parts, including hair, umbilicus, fingers, toe nails, and so forth.	—

INDEX

Page numbers in boldface type indicate the page on which the main discussion of the entry can be found.

ALSO AVAILABLE

Guidelines for Perinatal Care, co-authored by the American Academy of Pediatrics and the American College of Obstetricians and Gynecologists, focuses on a coordinated approach to infant care from conception through the postpartum and neonatal periods, 1983, 288 pages, $25.00.

Sports Medicine: Health Care for Young Athletes, was written by the Committee on Sports Medicine. The book includes discussions on such topics as assessing the athletic potential of children, nutrition, stress reduction, the role of physicians and athletic trainers, and the prevention and management of sports-related illnesses, injuries, and rehabilitation, 1983, 326 pages, $15.00.

Report of the Committee on Infectious Diseases, 19th edition, is written by experts in the field of infectious diseases and provides updated information on the control, prevention, and treatment of infectious diseases encountered in the Americas, 1982, 379 pages, $15.00.

School Health: A Guide for Health Professionals, 1981, was written by the Committee on School Health. The book discusses the role of school health programs and describes how these programs fit into the overall school program. Also discussed are ways in which parents, school officials, nurses, and physicians can work as a coordinated school health team, 1981, 297 pages, $15.00.

- -

Title	No. of copies
Guidelines for Perinatal Care @ $25.00	_____
Sports Medicine: Health Care for Young Athletes @ $15.00	_____
Report of the Committee on Infectious Diseases, 19th ed. @ $15.00	_____
School Health: A Guide for Health Professionals, 1981 @ $15.00	_____
UPS Shipping, add $1.60 each book	_____

TOTAL ENCLOSED $_____

Make check payable to:

**American Academy of Pediatrics
P.O. Box 1034, Evanston, Illinois 60204**

☐ AAP member
I.D. # (required for processing)_____ ☐ Non-member

Name _____

Address _____

City_____ State_____ Zip _____

MasterCard/Visa accepted. For charge orders call 1-800-323-0797.

Allow 3 weeks for delivery